C000083882

STONE AGE DIET

STONE AGE DIET

LEON CHAITOW

RECIPES BY ALKMINI CHAITOW

An OPTIMA book

© Leon Chaitow 1987

First published in 1987 by
Macdonald Optima, a division of
Macdonald & Co. (Publishers) Ltd

A BPCC PLC company

All rights reserved

No part of this publication may be reproduced,
stored in a retrieval system, or transmitted,
in any form or by any means without the prior
permission in writing of the publisher, nor be
otherwise circulated in any form of binding or
cover other than that in which it is published
and without a similar condition including this
condition being imposed on the subsequent
purchaser.

BRITISH LIBRARY CATALOGUING IN PUBLICATION DATA

Chaitow, Leon
  Stone Age diet.
  1. Nutrition
  I. Title
  641.1   TX353
  ISBN 0-356-12328-6

Macdonald & Co. (Publishers) Ltd
3rd Floor
Greater London House
Hampstead Road
London NW1 7QX

Photoset in 11pt Century by
🅰 Tek-Art Limited, Croydon, Surrey.

Printed and bound in Great Britain by
Hazell Watson & Viney,
a BPCC PLC company,
Aylesbury, Bucks

Illustrated by Alan Saunders

I wish to thank my wife and co-author Alkmini for her contribution to the section of this book which deals with the preparation of game and wild vegetables. She has a feel for food and cooking which is instinctive. This book is dedicated to her, and to my dear friend Alecos Kazantzis, who first drew my attention to the research work on Paleolithic diet. Now that the book is completed perhaps we can play golf again.

Differences between the dietary patterns of our ancestors, and the patterns now prevalent in industrialized countries, appear to have important implications for health. Physicians and nutritionists are increasingly convinced that the dietary habits adopted by Western society over the past 100 years make an important contribution to coronary heart disease, hypertension (high blood pressure), diabetes and some kinds of cancer. These conditions have emerged as dominant health problems in the past century, and are virtually unknown among the few surviving hunter-gatherer populations, whose way of life and eating habits most closely resemble those of pre-agricultural human beings (people of the Stone Age).

DOCTORS S. BOYD EATON AND MELVIN KONNER

CONTENTS

INTRODUCTION

A vegetarian for over 25 years, I had convinced myself of the superiority of this diet, at least in health terms. Social difficulties aside, it gave me a safe and sure sense of 'doing the right thing'. It was ecologically and economically sensible, with proper respect for humanitarian ideals. And it was indeed healthier than eating conventional modern food.

The revelation that this was not the only 'right' way of eating struck me like a bombshell when I read the research work of Doctors S. Boyd Eaton and Melvin Konner on Paleolithic diets.[1] Subsequent research, incorporating the findings of numerous other distinguished scientists, and my own observations over 30 years' clinical experience using nutritional methods in healing, lie behind the writing of this book.

Of particular value has been the research of two men whom I am proud to call friends: Professor Emeritus Emanuel Cheraskin and Professor Jeffrey Bland. Their books have enlightened me to the scientific aspects of what had been largely empirical knowledge, namely that diet and disease are inseparable.[2] If not always a causal factor, diet is always involved. Scientific evidence leads to the overwhelming and inescapable conclusion that there are at least two 'right' ways of eating in terms of the biological and physiological requirements of the human body: the vegetarian diet and the Stone Age diet.

The current state of health in the civilized world is extremely alarming, with a virtual epidemic of chronic degenerative diseases such as cancer, coronary heart disease, diabetes, mental illness and arthritis. Yet there are, and were, groups of people and entire periods of history free of these diseases. Many are absent or limited in vegetarian peoples, and they are not found among people currently living a Stone Age, hunter-gatherer way of life. They were almost totally absent in the Stone Age.

The World Health Organization, the American Senate Select Committee on diet, and the National Advisory Committee on Nutritional Education in Britain (NACNE), have all spelled out the strategy required to reduce chronic disease. Many of their recommendations are identical, or closely similar, to the dietary provisions of Stone Age people.

Stone Age diet, with its high contents of game meat, absence of refined carbohydrates, high fibre intake and other attributes, provides the human body with all its requirements, without the imbalanced ratios of essential nutrients which characterize modern eating habits. A major reason for this is the staggering difference in both the type and amount of fat between game and domesticated animals. Another is that the Stone Age diet excludes almost all dairy produce, while including large amounts of vegetable foods to compensate for the acidity of the high protein intake from game or fish. Also the high and varied fruit content of the Stone Age diet means a large consumption of vitamin C, but a minimal intake of sugar, salt and cereals. Our ancestors on this diet were taller and healthier than their agricultural descendants. This is equally true for the small number of people with Stone Age lifestyles today.

Numerous other researchers have contributed pieces to the mosaic which reveals the alternative to vegetarianism. Among these are Linus Pauling, the double Nobel prize winner; Herbert Shelton, pioneer nutritionist; Rudolph Ballentyne MD, researcher and

author; Sir Robert McCarrison, pioneer nutritionist;
M. Bircher-Benner, Swiss pioneer of nutritional methods
in healing; Melvin Page and Weston Price, whose studies
of human dental health have revealed so much about
nutrition; Dr William Kelley with his investigations into
metabolic variations in humans; Professor Roger
Williams and his definitive work on biochemical
individuality; Lawrence Dickey MD and his clinical
ecology studies; Lyall Watson for his investigation of
African traditions; and Robert Ardrey and Desmond
Morris for insights into prehistory.

All these, and others quoted in the text, deserve
recognition and thanks. Without them I could not have
pieced together a story which begins at the very dawn
of man, describing the fascinating circumstances in which
the original vegetarian mode became a hindrance rather
than an asset and showing how human survival has
hinged upon our dual biological potential.

Out of this comes a series of choices, which can bring
us all better health, less disease and a realization of the
potential which destiny has granted us.

LEON CHAITOW
Corfu 1986

1.
OUR BIOLOGICAL BLUEPRINT

Cancer will affect one adult in three in the USA and Western Europe by the end of the century. Coronary heart disease and strokes will kill or invalid one person in three in the industrialized world, many still in their prime.

Children are developing cancers at an alarming rate. Heart disease, in the form of atherosclerosis (arterial damage and blockage) is present in most young American and European children before they leave school.

Allergies, diabetes, respiratory and digestive problems, and symptoms ranging from premenstrual tension to migraines and hyperactivity in children have all been directly linked to nutritional patterns.

Yet all these conditions can be helped by adapting our diet, either to vegetarianism, or to the Stone Age diet (which includes game-meat and fish), both of which accord with human biological potential. It may even be that life expectancy itself can be lengthened to approach the limit decreed possible by genetic programming, that is, around 110 years. Certainly the quality of life can be enhanced immeasurably by freeing the latter years of life from the dread of illness and incapacity.

Diet alone is not the cause of all these conditions, but it is a major element, and the one we can do most about.

THE STONE AGE CONNECTION

What was the physique of our Stone Age ancestor, living in Europe some 30,000 years ago? If the imagination conjures up a hairy, half-stooped, ape-like individual, this is completely false.

Skeletal remains show that before people settled into an agricultural existence, when they were still hunter-gatherers, they were a full 15cm taller than their descendants 20,000 years later. These descendants, whose dietary pattern had altered as a result of the Neolithic revolution with its farms, towns, and settled way of life, were markedly inferior in physique.

As in Europe, so in North America. About 10,000 years ago, the indigenous people were big game hunters, and only began cultivating the land shortly before the arrival of the European colonizers. These settled native

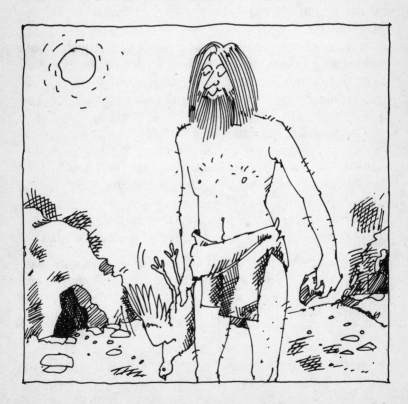

Americans had an inferior diet and were as a result much smaller than their hunting predecessors.

Modern humans are growing taller, but we still have not reached the full size of our free-living ancestors. It is our diets, so very different from theirs, that lie at the root of those diseases which have been described as 'affluent malnutrition', or 'the undernutrition of overconsumption'.[3]

TEETH AND HEALTH

One of the most accurate monitors of health is the state of a person's teeth. Teeth in fossil remains might appear diseased because simple wear and tear exposed the pulp cavity, but decay is hardly ever found in teeth from Neolithic times before man started farming. However decay is commonly found in the teeth of fossils belonging to the period after the start of agricultural settlements.[4]

Examinations of the skulls of early man found in South Africa and Java, and of prehistoric Maoris, native Americans and Eskimos, show a very low incidence of dental decay, with caries evident in only about 1%. In contrast, recent British reports show that 81% of five-year-olds entering school in Staffordshire had tooth decay; in Scotland 50% of three-year-olds and 95% of school leavers had tooth decay; and in 1963 5,440 full sets of upper and lower dentures were supplied to young people of 20 and under.

Melvin Page, dental surgeon, has described the relationship between diet, teeth, and general health.[5]

'Dentine, the bony structure of teeth, depends for its well-being upon its nourishment. If it is not well nourished, it is soft; if it is well nourished, it is hard and dense and resistant to bacterial invasion ... Man is a mechanical genius, and in this lies his undoing. He has been able to change his environment by his ingenuity, and by environment is meant not only his surroundings but his food. The character of his food has completely changed, and has changed to his disadvantage. The mechanical and chemical equipment of his body is no different now than it was 1,000 or 10,000 years ago. Nutritional changes which he has forced upon himself have led to the rapid rise of the degenerative diseases which constitute the major cause of death today.'

The shape of the jaw, and so the crowding or otherwise of the teeth, can also be affected by dietary changes. In a series of dramatic photographs, Dr Weston Price has shown the difference between people of the same tribe, when their diets altered towards 'civilized' patterns.[6] Those on a natural native diet of fish, game, roots, stems, leaves, berries, grains and peas have fine facial bone structures, wide dental arches and sound teeth. Those who have begun to eat refined, manufactured foods (canned foods, white flour, sugar) produce children with decayed teeth, narrow arches, deformity of the facial bones and narrowing of the air passages.

The same pattern is repeated among New Zealand Maoris and Eskimos, and also among the inhabitants of the Island of Harris off the Scottish coast. Dr Price's photographs show two brothers from this island, one living on a natural diet of locally available foods, and the other on white bread, marmalade and canned food. There could be no more dramatic contrast. Price tells us that the healthy brother ate chiefly oat products and sea foods, including a wide variety of fish and generally, no dairy products. Oat grain was the only cereal that could be matured satisfactorily in that climate. Some green foods were available in the summer and some vegetables grown and stored for the winter. This diet contained a liberal supply of fish, including the fish livers.

The once legendary health of the Scots is now one of the worst in the world. It has the highest incidence of heart disease in Britain, which in turn has the worst record in Europe. Dental health in Scotland is also appalling, as is the dietary pattern, with the Scots having the lowest intake of fresh vegetables and fruit per person in the United Kingdom.

FOOD FOR THOUGHT

Dr Price made a further dramatic finding. The deformity of the dental arch and the malformation of the facial bones was accompanied by lower IQs, personality disturbances, higher incidences of degenerative diseases such as tuberculosis, and also of birth defects.

It would be an oversimplification to say this is all because of dietary changes, but that there is some connection seems beyond doubt.

OTHER BONE DISEASES

There is no fossil record of deficiency diseases of the bone such as rickets before farming began to be practised in late Neolithic times. On the other hand osteoarthritis is found in all species of animals, including human beings. It is evident in the fossils of prehistoric reptiles and dinosaurs, and was common in early humans.

The main cause was not nutritional lack, but trauma and injury. Falls and bruising are triggers for such bone changes, and these were frequent with the intense physical activity of hunting and surviving in Paleolithic times.

Aside from what we can tell by examining the condition of the teeth and bones of fossil remains, there is little evidence of what diseases, if any, affected people in the Stone Age. The best indicator is the health of the people who have continued that way of life and diet.

HUNTER-GATHERERS TODAY

Before the agricultural revolution (about 10,000 years ago) the population of the world was 100% hunter-gatherer. Today this nomadic way of life is followed by only 0.01% of the population of the planet. This nevertheless still involves some 400,000 people, a large enough number for scientific investigation and assessment. It is about the same number as existed in the sixteenth century, when they represented 1% of the world population.

Eskimo hunter-gatherers do not develop rickets. They do so, however, when they abandon this way of life, settle in communities and start to eat Western-style food. Coronary heart disease is virtually unknown among free-living Eskimo people. Doctors working with Eskimos and native Americans state that, in 35 years no sign of malignant disease was seen among those following a traditional diet, whereas those on modern diets often required surgery for cancer, gall bladder disease, kidney, stomach and appendix problems. Tuberculosis is also common in the latter group.

The effects of different diets on the condition of the teeth of Eskimos and Indians

Percentage of diseased teeth	on traditional diet	on mixed diet*	on modern diet
Eskimos	0.15% caries	6.3% caries	21.1% caries
Native Americans	0.1% caries	25.5% caries	40.0% caries

*Mixed diet is part modern, part traditional

Teeth which had been worn down from chewing leather to soften it frequently showed damage right down to the pulp chamber. However, in time, these often filled with secondary dentine.

The traditional diet of these peoples comes mainly from sea animals and is also surprisingly rich in plant life.

THE BUSHMEN

Closer to the popular image of the hunter-gatherers of old are the still surviving African Bushmen. The concept of their life being a constant struggle for survival is completely wrong.

They choose their way of life knowingly, having every opportunity to settle, rear stock and cultivate the land. But this lifestyle, they feel, is likely to be less stable, and more stressful and precarious, than the nomadic way of life of their ancestors. Many modern farmers would probably agree.

17

If the population is small enough, in a hunter-gatherer environment, then the living is not difficult. The San Bushmen, of South Africa, are probably the best known, and have lived in the same area for a very long time. These people are artists of some merit, and their skeletons have been discovered in caves containing delicate rock paintings and some extraordinary carved bones. These bones, some 50,000 years old, have carefully engraved notches carved into them, and are thought to be calendar sticks, similar to the knotted strings of the Inca people of South America.

Rock paintings show images of people with the characteristic large and unusual buttocks of the Bushmen, alongside pictures of hunting equipment and animals. Some have been signed with the imprint of a hand dipped in pigment, identifying the artists as Bushmen, as the hands are notably small, like those of the modern Bushmen hunter-gatherers.

Present day Bushmen have a more stressful life than did their ancestors, since their area of operation has been limited by the encroachment of other peoples, notably the Bantu and the Whites of South Africa. Nevertheless they are demonstrably healthier than their peers, who have settled and altered their diets accordingly.

The Nomadic Bushmen have kept to their traditional way of eating: game, wild fruits, nuts, berries, bulbs and roots, and what honey can be found are the staples. They drink no animal milk, and their digestive system cannot tolerate it. They do, however, continue to breastfeed their young for up to four years, a common practice among hunter-gatherer people worldwide. Their salt intake, about two grams per day, is extremely low.

Cancer, high blood pressure, dental caries, mental illness and peptic ulcers are all unknown. Their health is infinitely better than that of most people living an urban European life.

THE HAZDA OF TANZANIA

The Hadza are completely nomadic, living in a semi-arid area of central Tanzania. Their unique language, related to that of the click language of the Bushmen of South Africa, prevents them from intermingling with neighbouring settled tribes, and they remain unaffected by civilization. They live in makeshift shelters and move on when the whim takes them. There are no signs of leadership among their groups, which break up when some want to go one way and others another. New individuals or groups join together whenever they meet by chance. In cases of disagreements which cannot be simply solved, the parties just separate and go their own ways.

Because they have never been short of food, they store none, and although considerable effort is required, they can always locate adequate supplies. As with the Southern Bushmen the men hunt, while the women gather fruits, berries, nuts and roots. Honey is prized, and much discomfort is endured in its recovery. It is eaten with the beeswax and the grubs.

The health of the Hadza is superb. There are no signs of malnutrition, nor of any of the diseases so common among their settled neighbours. Their one weakness appears to be a susceptibility to infection if wounded.[7]

THE MASAI

Tribes such as the Masai, Samburu, and Karamajong of Africa all live similar lives and have similar diets, with one notable exception. The Masai consume milk mixed with fresh blood, both taken from their nomadic herds of cows. Nutritionally the mixture of milk and blood is thought to provide them with essential oils, absent in milk, which is never drunk alone. They also eat abundant fruit, berries and other vegetation. They have remarkable physiques and health.

Nomadic peoples in Australia, South America, and other remote areas also bear witness to the fact that hunter-gatherers are well nourished, emphatically superior in health to those who have settled, and patently devoid of the diseases which kill most people in industrialized societies.

They also demonstrate artistic and cultural development which, in its own way, is as complex as our own. They are happy, well adjusted and intelligent.

WHAT HUNTER-GATHERERS EAT

The diets of the hunter-gatherer societies which remain are far more varied than might be imagined.[8] Even Eskimos include in their diets a great deal of plant food, mostly from lichen, kelp (seaweed) and berries such as cranberries.

Hunter-gatherers in general eat more plant than animal food, though they like meat and seafood when it is available.[9] They have a high fibre content in their diets, take no salt or alcohol, and never eat concentrated sugar save what honey they can scrounge.

The Eskimo people, from whom science has recently learned much about longchain polyunsaturated essential fatty acids, have a diet of dried salmon, seal oil, fish eggs, caribou meat, ground nuts, kelp, berries, flower blossoms and sorrel grass (preserved in seal oil), organs of large sea animals, and layers of whale skin (very rich in vitamin C). They have been found to eat some 24 different kinds of mosses and lichens, including cloudberry, barberry, crowberry, reindeer moss, and other Arctic plants.[10]

The Bushmen eat meat as and when it can be caught, along with birds, locusts, nuts, bulbs, fruits and berries. The nut of the Mangety tree (*ricinodentron rautenii*) provides protein when meat is in short supply. Insects of various sorts supplement the diet, ants being especially prized. Water is scarce, so they depend on the juices of fruits and bulbs such as the Tsamma melon. Recent studies of Bushmen in the Kalahari desert show that 19 days of hunting and gathering provided food supplies sufficient to last 100 days. Their daily calorie intake of some 2400 calories is higher than the European adult's average.

The nomadic Hadza eat a variety of animal meat. Importantly they attach little value to that part most eaten in the West, muscle meat. They eat everything, apart from the bones and the hide. They also eat a wide selection of fruits, seeds and roots.

It is worth noting that carnivores such as lions do not immediately eat the muscle regions of their prey. First they eat the intestines which provide them with the partly digested plant food contained there. They then consume the liver, spleen and kidneys, before going on to the lungs and heart. The ribcage bones are eaten next and only then, if they are not yet satisfied, are the muscles devoured.

This pattern is also followed by hunter-gatherer people and ensures a high intake of vitamins and such nutrients as iodine found in animal livers. Much animal fat is consumed, but of a different type to that found in domesticated animals (see below).

WHAT STONE AGE PEOPLE DID NOT EAT

Over the past 40,000 years there have been few genetic changes to our constitutions or digestive capabilities. The development of agriculture is too recent to have produced any major alteration. One change which is recognized, however, is the partial ability of human adults to digest the lactose in animal milk. The enzyme lactase, required for this, is present in infants in order for human milk to be digested.

Only a few groups, notably certain Northern Indian peoples, Northern Europeans, and some Africans (mainly from Uganda) are able to digest animal milk in any degree as adults. Orientals, most people of African descent, most Southern Europeans and about one in five Northern Europeans are unable to digest milk or milk products in any quantity. For these people milk drinking often results in bowel disturbances and flatulence. Allergies are also commonly related to dairy produce.

Doctors of clinical ecology (which deals mainly with allergy problems) are particularly concerned with the degree of adaptation to other foods which have been introduced to humankind relatively recently. Cereals in particular come under special scrutiny, since many individuals are sensitive to certain grains. Cereals and milk played no part in the Stone Age diet, at least not until Neolithic times.

Surprisingly, fish too was largely absent from the Stone Age diet until about 20,000 years ago. Before then few shells or fish bones are to be found in the debris of food refuse which litters many prehistoric sites.

STATURE

Early humans derived at least 50% of their energy from plant foods and the rest from meat.[11] Population growth, overhunting and climatic changes caused a gradual decline in this pattern, as more plant-based food and seafood was consumed, at the expense of meat, with a gradual introduction of agricultural produce.

Some 30,000 years ago humans were at the peak of their hunting skills and were consuming a diet rich in game and wild-growing plant foods of excellent quality. They were a full head taller than their farming descendants 20,000 years later. This probably reflects protein-calorie deficiency in the farming Stone Age diet. Such deficits make the individual not only smaller in stature, with skeletal evidence of inadequate nutrition, but also more susceptible to illness and infection.

John Robson MD of the University of South Carolina suggests that the abandonment of wild fruits as a dietary component may be responsible for many of the present day problems of modern man.[12] He notes that when people abandoned the hunter-gatherer way of life, the variety of foods decreased, and the intake of fruits and berries in particular was halved. The quality of the meat eaten also declined.

WHAT STONE AGE PEOPLE ATE

Paleolithic people were fond of meat from ungulated herbivores, that is, animals which themselves eat plant foods. There is little evidence of them consuming carnivorous animals such as lions. Omnivorous animals such as pigs were eaten, both after the farming revolution and in the wild state. Food remains in ancient sites include the bones of deer, bison, bear, early horse, mammoth and boar, all of which were commonly hunted. One bison carcass would provide an average of 1,500 kilos of meat, sufficient for many days of feasting for a hunter band. The fat content of such animals would also provide months of fuel for lamps.

With the Stone Age population of Europe probably no more than 100,000 people, and with wildlife plentiful, food shortage presented no problems. Hippopotami, which roamed Europe and were even found in Britain, could provide a full 3000 kilos of meat. In general animals which travelled in herds were selected for hunting. The separation of young or injured animals was a favoured technique of hunter-gatherer groups. Birds of many varieties were also hunted or trapped.

Eaton and Konner estimate the Stone Age daily energy intake at 3000 calories, about one-third from meat and the remainder from plant foods.[13] On a good day, after a successful hunt, a Paleolithic warrior might have been expected to eat a little over two kilos of food (2250 grams), of which at least 790 grams would be meat. The intake of calories from meat was five times that of modern Americans. Despite the high meat consumption, however, there was vastly less saturated fat although overall cholesterol intake was much the same.

The calcium intake was very high, in spite of the total absence of dairy products. Skeletal remains and the bones of modern hunter-gatherers show that calcium was never in short supply, as it now is in almost epidemic proportions in post-menopausal women in the West.

Fibre consumption was much higher than in the modern diet, which has implications for the prevention of cancer of the bowel and coronary heart disease.

Hardly any salt was consumed, only about a sixth of modern American consumption, and only a third of that recommended by health authorities today. The Paleolithic intake of vitamin C was extremely high, nearly five times greater than the modern Western average. Iron and folic acid were also plentiful.

Most importantly the type of fat consumed was predominantly polyunsaturated, as compared to the high modern intake of saturated fats. This is largely because game fat has uniquely different qualities and proportions from that in domesticated farm animals.

Whether we are concerned with atherosclerosis, coronary heart disease, cancer, diabetes, high blood pressure, diverticulitis, colitis or other conditions, these differences are important – for it is possible to minimize the risks of developing such diseases by altering our dietary pattern to accord with the Paleolithic diet (and, equally, vegetarianism).

THE STONE AGE CONNECTION – MYSTERY AND CLUES

Every good mystery has its share of clues. The secrets buried in our past are divined and illuminated by tiny, often apparently meaningless clues. Slivers and fragments of bones become, in the hands of the skilled paleontologist, readily interpretable documents. From these, whole bones have been reconstructed to reveal the posture abilities and gait of early humans. This is especially true of the fragments from key bones such as the pelvis, jaw or skull.

Bones often carry on them the imprint of the soft tissues to which they were once attached. From these a veritable science has grown, by which the flesh can literally be put back on the bones. Thus we now know what our forebears looked like, what they were capable of doing, and to a large extent, what they actually did. We can be fairly sure about what they were designed to eat and, with the evidence of food and tool remains found at prehistoric sites, also about what they did actually eat. Social habits, artistic and manufacturing abilities, and even beliefs have been discerned from the records uncovered.

By combining the skills of paleontologists, anthropologists, zoologists and other scientific disciplines, we can now look with confidence at a reasonable likeness of early human beings, and their even more distant ancestors who once walked the earth we have inherited.

FROM APE TO ASTRONAUT

The story of this book is our journey, over several million years. From ape to astronaut.

Tentative conclusions have been reached on the pattern of evolution from which the modern human (*homo sapiens*) has derived, though there are disagreements on details and gaps in our knowledge. Such areas of controversy between experts are of little significance to the main theme of this book. Whether *homo sapiens* came from one or other branch of the hominid line, or which type of *australopithecus, gracilis* or *robustus* was more closely related to human beings, is important to the anthropologist and paleontologist, but does not alter the facts of our dietary progression.

It is clear that the *australopethicines* (Southern apes) are a key stage in primate evolution. While the brain capacity of these humans/apes was relatively small (around 700cc) they had many characteristics which link them with us. Overlapping their period of activity was the near human, known as *homo erectus* (or 'upright') with a much larger brain of around 1,000cc.

Nearer to our own time we find both early *homo sapiens* ('wise man') and the Neanderthal people. Their brains ranged in size from 1,300 to 1,650cc for the Neanderthal to between 1,100 and 1,700cc (for early *homo sapiens*).

Neanderthal people (named from the valley in

Germany where their skeletal remains were first discovered in the 19th century) were highly intelligent, as were the descendants of *homo erectus*, the Cro-Magnon people discovered in France. They appeared some 40,000 years ago, and were in all senses modern humans. It is mainly these people we are speaking about when we refer to the Stone Age, though we should keep in mind a generalized picture of an evolving human with, in the latter stages especially, very little physical or intellectual difference from ourselves, apart from cultural and educational variations.

Here, then, is our biological blueprint. By eating what nature intended, those foods which we are genetically programmed to eat, digest and metabolize, as evidenced by our Stone Age ancestors, we can receive one invaluable ancestral gift — better health.

LIFE EXPECTANCY

One thing is certain about Paleolithic times: there was no overcrowding. Until agriculture began some 10,000–12,000 years ago, and people for the first time crowded into towns, many infectious diseases were extremely rare.[14] Tuberculosis is only known from the late Stone Age, and not at all in the Paleolithic times.[15] Malaria, too, is believed only to have started with agriculture as forests were cleared and pools created for the mosquitoes to breed in.[16]

But if there was less disease, the environment held other dangers. Fossilized remains often show evidence of violent death, and many of the skeletons are of relatively young people. Any injury, however slight, would severely handicap an individual when confronted by predators of supreme agility and viciousness. Defended only by their own relative agility and quick wits (though precious little speed or strength when compared with a sabre-toothed tiger) early people had to be in optimum mental and physical condition to stand much chance.

Conclusions about life expectancy based on fossil

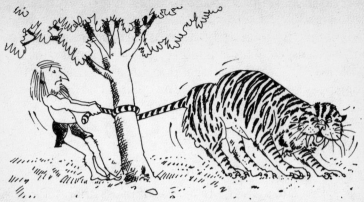

remains are not reliable, but leaving aside the question of vulnerability to attack by wild animals, there was probably a shorter overall life expectancy in prehistoric times.

THE GENES DICTATE

A shorter lifespan in prehistory seems to have been the result of genetic programming. Genetically speaking, there is little advantage to the species as a whole in individuals living longer. What is best for the gene, in its task of reproducing itself, is not necessarily what is best for the individual.[17]

The noted mathematical biologist, Gerald Hirsch, believes that in species which continue to reproduce until the end of their lives, life expectancy continues up to the point at which major disadvantages begin to accrue, that is when mutations begin to be noted in the DNA.[18] In humans, however, life continues long after reproductive activity ceases to have potential for producing new life, because human offspring require the presence of mature adults for them to grow and to be protected.

The maximum lifespan for humans has increased over the past several million years, and is currently estimated to be about 110 years. Dr Richard Cutler maintains that life expectancy has probably doubled during this time.[19] Over the past 100–200,000 years the rate of ageing has decreased and lifespan potential has increased by about ten years.

The relatively short lifespan of early humans was related both to genetic makeup and to lifestyle, but had nothing to do with nutritional factors. All the evidence supports the conclusion that they were healthier for the duration of their lives than we are today.

A LOOK INTO OUR PAST

If we attempt to look into the dim mists of the earth's past when our agile, more or less hairless ancestors were forced by malign climatic changes to scavenge for their food we may glimpse something of the way in which humans first deviated from nature's original nutritional blueprint. During this period they first learned the desirability and practical value of working together in groups to hunt and collect food and to protect themselves from the violent environment.

From a fruitarian background humans evolved through necessity towards an omnivorous pattern of eating. Their physiology was such that nature appears to have allowed for this deviation. This was indeed their salvation: the alterations which occurred in the climate, and so in food availability, were such that had they not been able to eat and digest meat, their extinction would have been assured.

Our Paleolithic ancestors followed a way of life dictated by circumstances, and they survived and ultimately thrived.

SEED FOR OUR FAMILY TREE

The records are incomplete, so the story of early human evolution from primordial ape to the modern day has gaps. These missing pieces of the puzzle lie in the realm of prehistory, so far back in time that it is difficult to comprehend in terms of its sheer antiquity.

It is not difficult for us to imagine events that occurred

a 100 or 200 years ago. We can relate them to the
generations of our family or to familiar places connected
by such events. But to contemplate a timescale which
stretches into hundreds of thousands and then millions
(and indeed tens of millions) of years brings a numbness
to the mind. Intellectually we may be able to build up
a reasonably accurate picture of early humans and their
way of life. Emotionally, however, it is very hard to relate
to people who, although ancestors, inhabited such dim,
dark spaces in the time continuum. But they lived and
breathed, struggled and loved, fought, feared and
suffered. These were not mere brutes, nor unthinking
hulks. They were sensitive, thoughtful, loving and
creative, often astonishingly so, given the opportunity.
If we can banish the barriers which time has created,
we can approach them with a feeling of compassion,
understanding and oneness. They were our grandparents,
uncles and aunts, and the world they lived in was this
world.

The extremes of climate and the struggle for survival
could be great, but the needs of men and women were
essentially the same then as now. The priorities were
the finding of food and shelter, the protection of the family
and the group with which it cohabited, the raising of
children and survival.

Nothing has changed except for the tools used to meet
these intrinsic needs. It is the tools which distinguish
them from us, which identify them as belonging to the
Stone Age.

THE DAWN OF HUMANITY

The physical split between apes and prehuman stock took
place some six million years ago. Fossil records are rare,
but become more plentiful from around four million years
ago. These show ape-like creatures called
australopithecines (Southern Ape).

These creatures walked on two legs, and critical
changes had already occurred in the pelvic and thigh

bones distinguishing them from apes proper and showing them as our forerunners, albeit considerably smaller. Now the hands were freed for uses other than locomotion. These liberated hands combined with the human brain were the dual sparks which lit the intelligence that would distinguish humanity.

The *australopithecines* split into two lines, *gracilis* and *robustus*. *Robustus* became extinct, while *gracilis* seems to have led to the modern human. *Homo erectus* was in evidence 1.6 million years ago, with bones being found as far afield as China.

By half a million years ago, *homo erectus* was using fire. This opened up the chance to alter and control the environment – to harden wood for weapons, to mould clay, to keep wild animals at bay, to cook meat, and ultimately to alter elements and create metal instruments and weapons.

Homo erectus had an upright posture, a large brain and, crucially, the ability to oppose the thumbs in holding and grasping movements. Skill and dexterity depend upon this, and only humans have this facility.

EXTINCT ANCESTORS

Nature, using the methods of natural selection, honed and refined the raw materials provided by the primate class to produce *homo erectus*. A variety of offshoots had also evolved which did not meet the exacting standards of the evolutionary process.

Australopithecus robustus was a large, heavy-boned creature, present until a million years ago. These gentle giants walked on two legs and had teeth and enormous jaw muscles which were clearly designed for vegetarian feeding. Dramatic alterations in their environment were to sweep them into an evolutionary dead-end, while their slimmer counterparts, called *gracilis*, would triumph over adversity because they were not restricted to a solely vegetarian pattern of feeding.

The highly intelligent Neanderthal human, unable to

cope with the demands of climatic changes, died out during the last Ice Age, which ended some 25,000 years ago. Cro-Magnon human and other examples of *homo sapiens* were already in existence, and thriving in a variety of habitats.

TECHNOLOGY

The making and using of tools is a central distinction between true humans and their ape-like predecessors. Chimpanzees will pick up and use a stick as a tool, often with some dexterity. They will not, though, patiently fashion one from raw material, such as stone. Stone Age humans, on the other hand, used stone with skill and sometimes great beauty to fashion useful implements. Their evolution is measured not so much by historical time, but rather by technical achievement.

The three major Stone Age periods are the Paleolithic (*paleo*, Greek for very old), Mesolithic (*meso*, Greek for middle), and Neolithic (*neo*, Greek for new). *Lithic* is from the Greek *lithos*, stone. These periods are not classified in terms of fixed dates. Rather they represent stages of technological progress. For example, in terms of their way of life and development, today's aborigines in Australia are Neolithic people. However, as has been clearly demonstrated, they are every bit as capable of operating a computer or composing music as is an

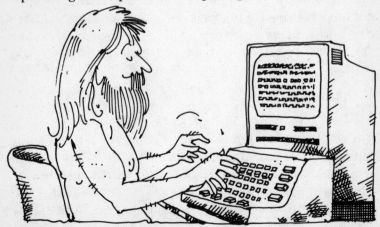

inhabitant of Chicago or Southend-on-Sea, given the education and training.

The human mind in the Stone Age had the same potential as our minds of today. Prior to the Stone Age, humans and their predecessors had been around for some 20 million years with little need for tools of any kind. Fruit and nuts were to be had in abundance, requiring little effort to gather. It was the need to adapt in order to survive which spurred our ingenious ancestors to improvize with the most plentiful material to hand, stone.

SURVIVAL DIET

Between 7½ and 4½ million years ago, a split took place, which sent apes in one evolutionary direction and humans in another. We know from the contents of ancient cave dwellings that by two million years ago both *homo habilis* and the dominant species *homo erectus* were using stone tools and had become meat eaters. The meat may have been scavenged, killed by large animal predators, or culled by hunting. The reason for the switch to an omnivorous (literally 'all devouring') diet was quite simple. It was a matter of survival.

Climatic changes meant that fruit in plenty was no longer available. Had humans not adapted to a varied pattern of eating, they (and therefore, we) would certainly not have survived to inherit the earth. Genetic alterations had, fortuitously or by design, endowed them with the dental and digestive equipment to process food other than fruits.

TRANSITION

The ability to fashion tools with which to cut and skin animals, as well as weapons with which to kill them, was a matter of necessity. The finding of trimmed stones in the proximity of animal remains in caves and among fossil deposits confirms the change of habits. The hunter had emerged. A harsh struggle for daily survival was now in progress.

The period of paradise may well have existed many epochs earlier, when the day's food supply could be had by plucking fruits from the trees. No tools were needed then. No clothing was required. The only blot was that humans themselves were distinctly edible.

Now climatic change brought a reduction in food, and so competition for it. Shelter, clothing and the means of killing and processing animals became essential.

From a jungle of plenty where the only danger was becoming a meal for a predator, our ancestors were forced to adapt to different habitats. In bush and scrub-filled landscapes, where they could better hunt their new found sources of food, they were also more vulnerable. For here, rather than in the thick jungle, was the natural hunting ground of the sharp-fanged, long-clawed, swift-footed natural killers. Tools were desperately needed to hunt with and for protection.

WHEN THE WEATHER WENT MAD

We are, regrettably, all too familiar with the TV portrayal of starving children in Africa and elsewhere, after several years when the rains have failed to come. Imagine not a few such dry years, nor even a few hundred, or thousand. Imagine – and it is far from easy – a period of millions of years when rainfall was reduced to about a quarter of the normal level. And imagine this happening after a period of millions of years of stable weather, resulting in the development of forms of life accustomed to plentiful and abundant vegetation.

For the first primates water was never in short supply and food was there for the eating. This was the situation throughout the Miocene era which lasted from about 24 million years ago until 5 million years ago. For the best part of that enormous timescale, the African seedbed of humanity was a paradise of plenty. Then slowly the rains decreased. The forests began to shrink and life became

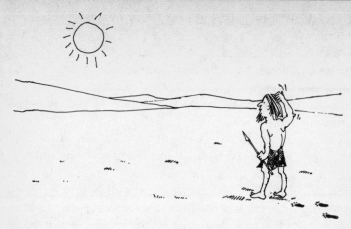

a struggle. This did not occur overnight but over tens of thousands of years. There was a gradual spread of grassland and scrub bush regions, with a slow encroachment of deserts until they claimed much of Africa.

Gone were many of the rivers and lakes. The residual forests in what is now the Congo could no longer support human life. Now, more than ever before, our ancestors found themselves a source of food for other, equally desperate creatures. Migration became an essential part of their survival. Agile, sharp-witted and hungry, they set off for distant parts.

THE SHAPING OF HUMANITY

The harshness of the Pliocene period marked a turning point for humanity. It was now that the ability to eat meat, and to digest it, was lifesaving.

Being creatures of social habits, humans lived in small groups. Compared to the predator ancestors of today's great cats, the lions, leopards and cheetahs of Africa, humans were puny. Their movement was pathetically slow, and only compensated for by cunning. Skill in weapon construction made up for the lack of claws and ripping teeth.

The planning of hunts, and communication within

groups, ensured enough meat for sufficient numbers to stay alive and keep the species in existence. Learning the skills of building traps, manufacturing tools and weapons, and organizing the hunt led to the evolution of a social structure, with a hierarchy of authority. Human society was born.

The drought went on for an incredible period of ten million years. The fossil records of this time are scanty. With no rivers to speak of, there was no damp clay or mud. There was also little rain, and therefore no deposition of lime to fossilize the remains of living creatures. The weather which inspired our evolution also ensured that no records of these changes would be left behind.

At the end of the Pliocene epoch, around two million years ago, the rains returned and the Pleistocene era began. Humans were now far more developed creatures as a result of this crucible of experience from which they had emerged. In the desperate battle for survival, for finding water and food, intelligence was the redeemer. The puny frame was saved by its brain.

In the Pleistocene epoch, the anatomical changes which characterize humanity were complete. The critical ability to use the hands in a more complex way than our ape-like ancestors spurred the intelligence available in the large human brain.

This was one of the central physical keys which unlocked the future once the upright posture had been perfected. Standing erect, and so turning the spine through a 90° angle, caused no little problem in terms of structural stability. In the words of Professor Irwin Korr, of Texas University College of Osteopathic Medicine, our spines are 'a perfect cantilever bridge which has been turned into an unstable skyscraper'.

THE ROLE OF THE SEXES

From the hunt, humans learned intelligent planning and strategy. Communication between co-operating

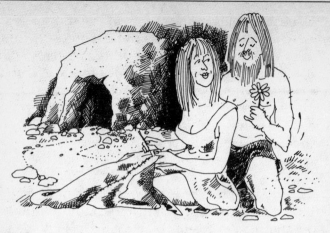

individuals was necessary, and this which encouraged the development of language. When the hunters were away food storage and forethought were necessary to protect the family group.

The roles of the sexes became more clearly defined as a result of the specialization of tasks. The care of the young was assigned to women, whilst the physically stronger males went in search of sustenance for the group. These changes were not merely cultural, but also biological, according to Desmond Morris.[20] They included pair-bonding, through the process of falling in love and remaining faithful to one partner, which was a distinct advantage to the evolving pattern of life of hunter-gatherer society.

This was contrary to normal primate behaviour, and reflected humanity's adaptation to new needs and circumstances. Yet is there something of the fall from grace, the leaving of the Garden of Eden, lying deep in the human unconscious? Is there still an echo in our minds of the wrenching departure from that safe, green, fruit-abundant paradise lost?

RACIAL ORIGINS

Here then were creatures moulded by climatic disaster, creatures forced into using their brains so as to become hunters, a role for which they were ill-equipped in terms of physique and previous experience. Yet they were not mere brutes. There are amazing records which testify to these same creatures' artistic talents, their enquiring minds and even to musical ability.

With the coming of the rains about one million years ago Africa became again a place of plenty. Animal and vegetable life prospered, and humans, no longer restricted to their ancient jungle home by their diet of fruits and nuts, wandered far afield. Evidence of human presence at this time has been found across the breadth of Africa and into Europe and Asia. The differences which resulted, in terms of colour, language and custom are part of the legacy we have inherited.

TOOLS AND THEIR SIGNIFICANCE

Our primitive ancestors were using tools two million years ago. The earliest ones found are almost indistinguishable from the natural stones. Once the stones began to be trimmed and shaped they became not only recognizable, but distinguishable in terms of their functions.

The earliest tools were pebbles, fashioned into rough choppers, the edge made by chipping off a few flakes from one side. These were used as weapons, and as tools for cutting meat and skinning the kill. The next leap forward came when, instead of striking one stone against another to make the cutting edge, humans learned to use a primitive form of chisel. By holding another stone, or a piece of bone or hard wood, against the surface to be worked, and striking this with a stone, the final product could be shaped more delicately, to produce a sharp pointed instrument with multiple uses.

The hand-axe, as this is called, was often a highly fashioned work of art, carefully and painstakingly formed into a pear or oval shape. As the flaking process became more skilful, the flakes themselves were found to be of value as knives and scrapers. One million years ago the

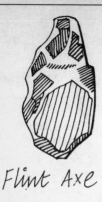

Flint Axe

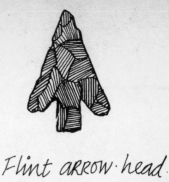

Flint arrow·head

floors of camp sites, caves and living areas were littered
with a variety of tools, and in particular with hand-axes.
Lyall Watson tells us 'the most mysterious and wonderful
thing about the hand-axe is that it is unnecessarily
beautiful. The delicacy and symmetry of its design, the
quality of the workmanship, and the time devoted to its
manufacture, all go beyond functional demand.'[21] The
evidence is that the artistic and creative forces of
humankind were emerging.

THE REFINING OF TOOLS

The first major development was this delicately worked
instrument, the hand-axe. Superbly efficient in
aerodynamics, it was the forerunner of more and more
advanced instruments. Early humans made knives,
weapons, borers and engraving tools. They made
harpoons and dart points out of bone, ivory and the antlers
of deer, and fine bone needles for sewing skin. Needles
were first in evidence around 16,000 BC. Now it became
possible to stitch the skins together; to sew water bags
and so create the opportunity for long journeys. Hides
sewn together were even used for primitive boat
coverings.

As the middle and late Stone Age periods passed, the
refinement of tools continued. Amongst the artefacts
discovered which date back to this period are tool handles,

arrow shafts, sledge runners, nets and objects made of birch bark.

THE DAY BEFORE YESTERDAY

By around 20,000 years ago humans had begun to exploit the sea. Fish played but a small part in the early Stone Age diet and economy, but by the late Stone Age there is evidence of consumption of the fruits of the sea.

In Neolithic times, the late Stone Age, people began to live in fixed settlements and towns. Agriculture had begun. Domestication of animals and the growing of crops were about to revolutionize the future of humanity. Now freed from the tasks of food gathering and hunting, humans had time for the development of culture, for the specialization of skills and for invention in the inexorable progression to modern times.

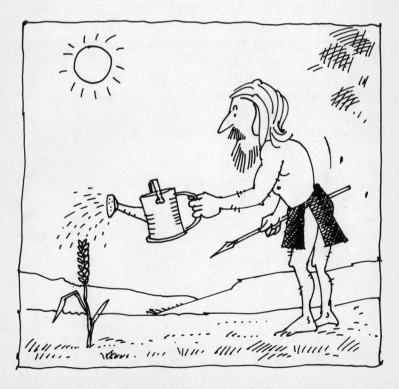

THE HUNT

We can picture how people of the Stone Age used cunning to overcome their physical inferiority in the hunt by looking at modern hunter-gatherer practice.

Lyall Watson gives us an example of how humans can, in certain situations, become highly specialized scavengers. The Hadza of Tanzania, for example, will sit watching the sky for the movement of vultures. When they see them spiralling down to eat, they follow them and, with a concerted screaming rush, drive them and any other scavengers or predators away. Acquiring a ready made meal would surely have appealed to the minimally armed humans of the early Stone Age, too. While forced to learn hunting, they were obviously also bound to gather or scavenge for whatever came to hand be it wild honey, bugs, grubs, edible roots or fruit.

More conventional in terms of our vision of the hunter is a rare find near Clacton in Southern England – a primitive lance made from yew wood which had been hardened by fire. A more complete lance, also of fire-hardened yew, was discovered in Germany. Nearly three metres long, it lay between the ribs of a long extinct elephant (*hesperoloxodon antiquus*). This brings to mind the hunting technique of modern pigmy tribesmen in Africa, who spear an elephant and then trail it until it falls from loss of blood.

Another technique employed was probably similar to that of Patagonian hunters who use rounded stone balls (*bolas*). Such worked stones have been found at prehistoric sites, and were probably hurled from a sling at smaller game. The balls would be attached to each other by thongs and the animals brought down by having them thrown at their legs.

Naturally occurring poisons were almost certainly used in killing animals for food. Such poisons are effective no matter which part of the animal is hit, so long as the skin is penetrated, and they present no hazard to the consumer.

ON THE MENU

The variety of animals found at sites in many countries reflect the wide choice open to our meat-eating early ancestors. In China, at Choukoutien, debris found dating back to 300,000 years ago included bones from the following: sabre-toothed tiger, leopard, hyena, elephant, rhinoceros, horse, bison, water buffalo, camel, wild boar, sheep, antelope and various types of deer.

If the drawings of animals on their walls reflect what our ancestors ate, then the 'cave of treasures' in the Dordogne region of France offers a bonanza: 150 mammoths, 26 bison, 14 goats, 12 rhinoceroses, 12 ibex, 6 snakes, 2 cats, an antelope, a deer and a bear. In one African site near the Olduvai Gorge the remains were found of meals of pig, antelope, horse and baboon, not to mention birds, rodents, snakes and frogs. It may not sound appetizing, but it was certainly nutritious.

'Were early humans cannibals?' This is an uncomfortable question which has been asked by some researchers. A number of human skulls have been found which had been opened from the base (at the *foramen magnum*), and it has been suggested that this method is necessary for the removal of the brain without splitting the skull open. This might have been either a ritualistic act or a cannibalistic one. Certainly, early humans must have been well aware of the tasty contents of the skulls of other animals, but whether they were cannibals we shall never know.

HOME LIFE AND CULTURE

Carleton Coon, describing one of the most primitive tribes on earth – the Tiwi of Australia – tells us: 'Had the Tiwi become extinct several centuries ago, there would be nothing much to indicate the heights of art this people reached, the fun they had or the sophistication of their way of life.'[22]

We must bridge the gap of time and remind ourselves

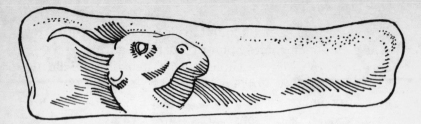

that there was everything from art to family arguments, from love affairs to games in Stone Age life.

Rock paintings of great antiquity show fine artistic outpourings, which may be symbolic, religious or simply painted for the pleasure of it. The effort which went into manufacturing tools and the beautiful results speak of a desire to create form and symmetry. And then there was music. One Neolithic instrument, the 'lithophone', an example of which has been found in Vietnam,

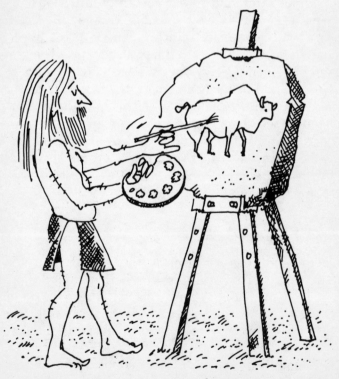

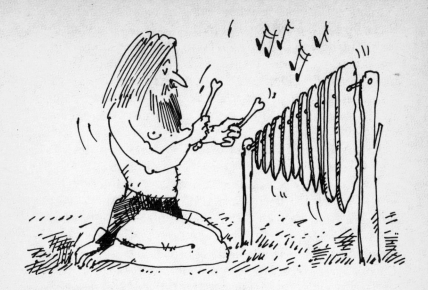

comprises ten stones carefully tuned, by chipping, to produce a musical scale.[23]

STONE AGE MINING

In the 19th century, during the boom years of the South African diamond rush, it was common knowledge among the diggers that if Stone Age tools were found amongst the earth and rock in which they were searching, there would be little purpose in continuing to look for diamonds. They would have been removed by ancient hands. In the early 1970s an earth-moving machine, having dug a wide ditch, cleared all the earth and gravel to the bed rock. At the bottom lay a number of fine Stone Age tools alongside piles of graded rock, with all the diamonds removed. Cut into the bedrock were engravings (probably fashioned with diamonds) of animals and a form of late Neolithic script appearing as a series of short lines, extending from a longer one.

Mining of hematite, a mineral consisting of iron oxide, was widespread. The red, earthy form of this mineral, known as red ochre, is used as a pigment, and there is

evidence of its use in burial rites in Neanderthal times.
Red ochre still plays a major part in African folk tradition,
for painting the body and face in ritual manners and in
the burial of the dead. Sites in Zambia indicate that
manganese dioxide, used for dying and colouring, was
also mined in the Stone Age. Recent finds, according to
Lyall Watson, indicate mining for pigments as far back
as 140,000 years ago.

The climatic changes of the Pleistocene era saw
widespread migration. Ice age was followed by dry
periods, wet periods and more ice. It is estimated that
in the whole of Africa south of the Sahara there were
no more than half a million people 50,000 years ago.
Thanks to migration there were larger numbers already
developing their own unique characteristics in Asia and
Europe. The route out was probably across from Africa
to Spain, a distance of under ten miles – when the sea
was at its lowest, only six miles.[24] The industry of hand-
axe manufacture spread from the Atlantic coast of North
Africa to the Bay of Bengal, and from the North Sea to
the Cape of Good Hope.

2.
THE VEGETARIAN OPTION

Any dietary pattern which aims to promote high levels of health should meet human genetic requirements. This is true both for the meat-eating hunter-gatherers, and for our original, fruit-eating, earliest ancestors.

There are in most societies people who have opted for a pattern of eating which takes them close to the diet which existed before the Miocene era. This is the vegetarian mode which attempts, knowingly or unknowingly, to duplicate the pattern of the dwellers of the forest, where vegetable-based foods were readily to hand, and health was superb.

When duplicated in modern society, this can lead to a higher level of well-being than that of conventional, meat-eating people, as long as the vegetarian is aware of nutritional requirements and avoids denatured, over-refined foods. There are a great many unhealthy vegetarians, without adequate protein intake, or who eat excessive refined carbohydrate.

MEAT OR VEG?

Having said that both vegetarianism and meat-eating, based on the Stone Age and earlier prototypes, are correct diets, there is nonetheless some argument about the nature of the early transition from one to the other.

Jon Wynne-Tyson insists that the view of our ancestors becoming omnivorous, and taking to flesh-eating en

masse, is incorrect.[25] He sees the meat-eating pattern
as a deviation from the norm of the fruitarian-vegetarian
mode. He argues eloquently for our physiological
similarity to the great apes and dismisses the views of
researchers such as Desmond Morris and Robert Ardrey,
who hold that the evolutionary branch of early man which
did tend to a vegetarian way of life failed to survive into
modern times. Wynne Tyson asserts that 'whatever
climatic or other chance of nature provoked a proportion
of our ancestors to take to the eating of animal flesh (a
change that might well have eliminated all but the more
adaptable), nothing in their physical structure was fitted
for such a drastic dietary shift.'

Indeed, many could not adapt to a hunting, scavenging
way of life. Many were insufficiently adapted to the
digestion and assimilation of meat. Equally, many
vegetarian ancestors fell by the wayside because they
could not adapt. Those that survived were the ones that
nature had provided with the genetic characteristics best
suited to the demands of change. This is what evolution
is all about. We may, by nature, be either vegetarian or
meat-eating. The choice is ours.

CONTRASTING VIEWS

Linus Pauling, double Nobel prize-winner, tells us, 'If
we lived on raw fresh plant foods, as our ancestors did
some millions of years ago, there would be no need for
concern about getting adequate amounts of the essential
foods, such as vitamins.'[26]

Nutritionist and author Herbert Shelton sees the
archetypal human as a frugivore, whatever adaptations
he has had to make along the way in order to survive.
'The number and structure of the teeth, the length and
structure of the digestive tract, the position of the eyes,
the character of the nails, the function of the skin, the
character of the saliva, the relative size of the liver . . .
and many other factors, all bear witness to the fact that
a human is constitutionally a frugivore.'[27]

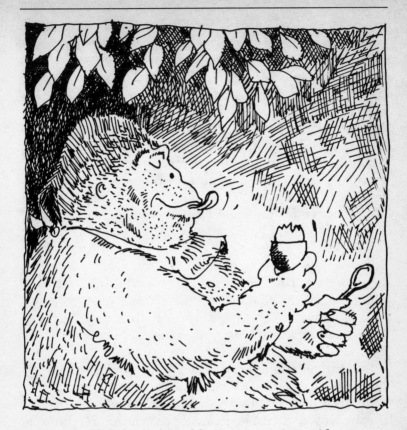

This is slightly disputed by more recent evidence on the behaviour of the great apes who are often thought of as pure frugivores. Desmond Morris explains: 'The ape's old forest diet was not all fruit and nuts. Animal proteins were undoubtedly of great importance . . . juicy bugs, eggs, young helpless nestlings, tree frogs, and small reptiles were all grist to the mill.[28] Coates confirms that the apes prize meat highly, and says that chimpanzees have been observed deliberately hunting.[29]

According to Eaton and Konner, the early humans were capable of adapting without much difficulty to a meat-orientated diet, and even from the Miocene era their fossilized dental remains seem suitable for mastication of both animal and vegetable material.[30]

The adaptation to meat, in Rudolph Ballentyne's view,

was accomplished with some difficulty.[31] He asks: 'How could an essentially peaceful food-gatherer learn the cunning and aggression necessary for stalking and killing prey? Those individuals (in whom) flesh foods stimulated a tendency towards aggressiveness and hunting would have a definite edge on their fellows, and would tend to survive and propagate.' He argues that as meat-eating became an integral part of human nature, the hunters would become aggressive and conquer more peaceable groups, and so become dominant. But when agriculture replaced hunting, they 'would suffer from a stimulation of aggressive feelings and hunting instincts, that would have no comfortable outlet in a settled peaceful community.'

The implications, in modern society, are that the repressed hunting instinct finds an outlet in violence, crime, terrorism, and on a national scale warfare. Thus, 'what had been a dual capacity for gathering or hunting, with great adaptive potential, could have now become a major danger for survival.'

Ballentyne points to the tradition in India, which prescribes a meat diet for the warrior castes and a vegetarian diet for the Brahmins, who dedicate themselves to spiritual advancement and study. Our dual biological potential is spelled out in this example. We may continue meat-eating (in a modified manner, using game), which would encourage the associated drives. These drives, if we are aware of them, may be channelled into creative pursuits, but if we are not, they may become destructive. On the other hand, we may decide that the adaptation to meat-eating no longer serves any practical purpose, and follow a vegetarian way of living, which leads us towards the original Miocene pattern of eating and a gentler, more philosophical nature.

Both meat-eating and vegetarian ways of life are in accord with our known biological potentials.

WHAT IS A VEGETARIAN?

George Bernard Shaw, a quintessential vegetarian, reminds us that 'a vegetarian is no more dependent solely on vegetables for sustenance, than is a Catholic dependent on cats'.

A vegetarian is one who avoids animal flesh, be this fish, fowl or meat. One who abandons all animal products is described as a vegan. This choice is fraught with potential hazards unless great care is taken in the selection of appropriate vegetable sources of protein. The vegan mode of eating satisfies certain philosophical requirements, but does appear to fly in the face of the behaviour of the great apes, for example, who do eat eggs and animal protein, when available.

A vegetarian pattern of eating, including some animal protein (eggs, etc.) but little if any dairy produce, and constructed according to rational guidelines, is a health-promoting one and in accord with the pre-Stone Age pattern.

METABOLIC TYPES

Attacking the lifestyle and eating pattern of meat-eaters demeans vegetarians, as does the belittling of vegetarianism by meat-eaters. Vegetarians are correct, and so are the eaters of meat, from the viewpoint of biological determinants. Nature has allowed for choice – or rather has provided an escape route – should one or other nutrient source become unavailable, or be undesirable. By what may be called 'metabolic typing', some individuals are shown to be better suited to a high-protein pattern, whereas others thrive when they become vegetarians.

Doctors William Kelley[32] and Henry Bieler[33] have sought to identify characteristics which are the outward signs of these variable metabolic types. There are seldom absolutely clearcut examples to be found, as most people are a mixture of several characteristics. If one of the patterns described below seems to fit you more closely than any of the others, the advice would be to follow the guidelines for that type and to assess the benefits.

MEAT-EATING TYPE

In general terms, the individual best suited to a diet high in animal protein is physically stocky, has curly hair, a low hair line and large teeth, which are extremely resistant to decay. Meat-eaters have a heavy jaw, dry warm skin, a short neck, broad chest, protuberant abdomen and thick or short fingers and toes with the moons of the nails being small or absent.

They have strong constitutions, powerful muscle-tone, and are seldom constipated. They are resistant to infection, seldom feel the cold and sleep well.

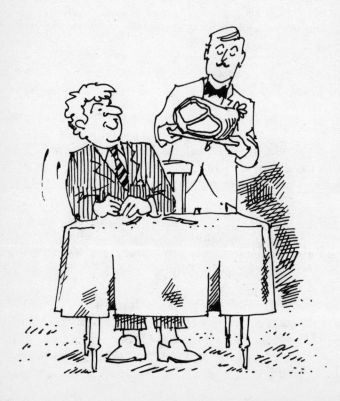

Meat-eaters have unlimited energy, warm personalities and are gregarious by nature, with a large circle of friends. Since their digestion and elimination is excellent, they cope well with high-protein foods.

The main danger is high fat content, derived from modern domesticated animals, causing degeneration of the cardiovascular organs and a tendency to become overweight. This can be minimized by using Stone Age meats.

VEGETARIAN TYPE

The vegetarian is often characterized by a large head, with a domed forehead. The joints are lax, often 'double jointed'. There may be a tendency to flat feet or knock knees. The moons on the finger nails tend to be well defined, and the teeth are unusually large. These individuals will often be very tall, with long limbs, and are frequently intuitive, with a dominant artistic or creative side.

They tolerate pain well and have strong sexual drive.

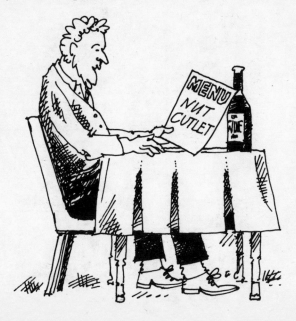

There is often a tendency to depend on stimulants such as alcohol or caffeine.

Lack of protein is a common vegetarian problem, best met by the inclusion of ample supplies from vegetable sources (nuts, pulses, grains, etc.), plus a little animal protein if desired.

THE MIXED-FEEDER TYPE

The individual who is neither a strongly defined meat eater nor an obvious vegetarian is the mixed feeder, and is often of delicate physical structure.

They have a thin body, long chest and neck, with finely made hands and shapely fingers. The teeth are small and narrowly spaced. Mixed feeders have expressive eyes, a fine silky head of hair but very little body hair. They have heightened sexuality, and the entire nervous system tends to be easily aroused. They are often dissatisfied, become easily fatigued and find concentration difficult. They wake early and refreshed, but dream a great deal.

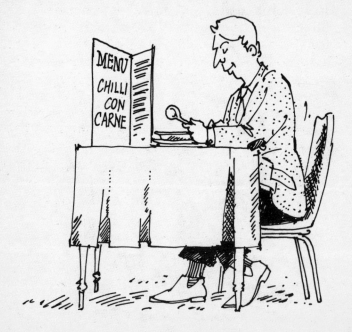

These individuals are capable of going either way in the dietary spectrum, functioning well on protein food derived from fish and fowl. They are sensitive to excessive salt intake.

WHY VEGETARIAN?

There are other reasons than metabolic type-casting for becoming a vegetarian.

Compassion for animal life seems to be a major element in the choice of many young people. But if they simply abandon meat and fail to take care of the protein requirements of the body, the new eating pattern is infinitely less desirable than the one previously followed.

The resources of the earth are limited, and the production of animal-based foods such as meat is extremely wasteful. Economically and ecologically the argument against meat consumption is strong. For every kilo of meat for the table, 7 kilos of cereal must have been consumed as animal feed. This cereal food could feed a family in Africa for two weeks. It can take up to 14 kilos of feed to produce a pound of beef or pork.[34]

In the 1960s the annual consumption of cereals in the USA had reached 862 kilos per head. But of course the American public were not consuming over two kilos of cereal per day. Over 90% of it went into meat production. The energy implications have been spelt out in *The Economist*: 'By the time mechanization, fertilizer, pesticides, transport, processing and supermarketing are added in, at least five units of energy (kilocalories) have been invested to produce one unit of energy in the consumer's actual diet.'[35]

The ecological argument against meat is summed up by Dr Kenneth Mellanby[36]: 'Not only do they (the livestock on Britain's land) use the grazing land of 29 million acres, but three-quarters of the acreage of tillage is sown with crops for livestock. In addition, many tons of animal feed are imported, much of it from countries

where human malnutrition and starvation are rife. When
we consume a large steak, we are eating something which
may have used enough grain to keep a family in drought-
stricken Africa for a week.'

The other argument against domesticated meat is, of
course, that of health.

GETTING ENOUGH PROTEIN

The amino acids which the body uses to build the
multitude of its protein-based component cells include
some ten different ones which are called 'essential amino
acids'. Meat or other animal protein contains the full
complement of essential amino acids, from which the body
can synthesize all others needed.

Plant proteins from individual sources (such as grains
or beans) have one or other of the amino acids missing.
To live healthily on plant food alone, an individual
requires a combination of sources, which together provide
all the necessary amino acids. For example a combination
of grains and pulses, eaten together, meets this
requirement.

Compared with more concentrated protein sources such
as meat or eggs, a greater bulk of plant food is required
in order to provide adequate protein. Dairy produce is
a source of protein, of course, for as with eggs or meat,
the animal has already done the synthesizing of the
protein from plant life. However, dairy produce has other
undesirable properties, which will be discussed in
Chapter 4.

The ultimate protein in our body cells is identical
whether it comes from meat or plants, as long as all the
amino acids are present. For the vegetarian who combines
pulses (anything from the bean family) and grains, or
nuts, or seeds (sunflower, pumpkin, etc.) there should
be no risk of protein deficiency, especially if eggs are
included in the diet.

OFFICIAL NUTRITIONAL GUIDELINES

In 1977 the McGovern Committee (Senate Select
Committee on Nutrition and Human Needs) issued a
document of 'dietary goals', which it maintained would
transform the health of the American nation, if
implemented. Anyone following the general guidelines
for vegetarianism (see recipe section) will automatically
be following the McGovern recommendations.

The report suggests, for example:

1. Increased carbohydrate consumption to account for
   55–60% of energy intake.

2. Reduced overall fat consumption, from current 40%
   to 30% of energy intake.

3. Reduced saturated fat consumption to account for 10%
   of total energy intake, balancing this with fats of
   polyunsaturated and monounsaturated origin.

4. Reduced cholesterol intake, to about 300 mg per
   day.

5. Reduced salt intake, by about 75%, to approximately
   3 grams per day.

Most of these guidelines automatically follow a change
to vegetarianism, and many follow a change to Stone Age
eating.

3.
WHATEVER HAPPENED TO MEAT?

Walter de la Mare expressed a basic truth in verse:

> It's a very odd thing
> As odd as can be
> That whatever Miss T eats
> Turns into Miss T.

In other words, we are what we eat.

There is ample evidence of the influence on health of hereditary factors. One of the most important researchers into this connection has been Professor Roger Williams.[37] In the study of the calcium requirements of just 20 students he found great variation in the amounts needed by each one to maintain calcium balance in the body, ranging from 222 milligrams to 1081 milligrams per day. This means that individual requirements differed by 400%. In larger sampling, Williams assures us, the variation between the greatest need and the least need would be even larger.

The same applies to all nutrients, whether minerals, vitamins, carbohydrates, proteins or fats. We are individually programmed as to our requirements, which again alter according to other circumstances, such as illness, pregnancy, extremes of climatic condition, stress, etc. This programming is genetically determined, and recommended intakes may be far too much, or too little, for some individuals. The chance of providing the exact requirements, so that optimum levels are achieved, is small, and this leads in many people to a state of health which is below what is possible.

So, Williams says, 'practically any human weakness, deformity, deficiency or disease can be combatted by supplying the needed nutrients to the right locality, at the right time. Conversely almost any deformity, weakness or disease could be created or accentuated by lack of a crucial nutrient, at a crucial time.'

We have inherited from our ancestors particular genetic characteristics, which may help explain the work of Kelley and Bieler in assessing the 'types' described in the previous chapter. If we are constitutionally inclined towards meat-eating, then this requirement should be met, as part of our biochemical individuality. But what sort of meat should be eaten?

WHAT MEAT?

Paleolithic people obtained their meat and other animal protein from wild animals, mostly from what are called gregarious ungulated herbivores, such as deer. The modern beef cow is of similar origins, and yet is considered undesirable. Why? One point is that our ancestors were more interested in the organs of the animal than in the muscle meat popular today.

The meat of wild game, whether fowl, venison, boar, or rabbit, is usually darker than that of domesticated animals. When the fibres of the meat are examined (under a microscope and after staining), the differences are striking. This relates directly to the difference in fat content and to the nature of the animal's activity when alive.

HOW MUCH FAT?

The fat content is the main difference between these meats. Wild animals have very little superficial fat, whereas domesticated animal meat contains fat, not only superficially around the tissues, but also in the actual fascial planes (the connective tissue covering the muscles), and as 'marbling' in the muscles.

The life cycle of a farm animal is quite different to that of a wild one. The objective of the farmer is to produce maximum non-fibrous muscle and bulk in the most tender form possible. It is not in the farmer's interests to have animals expending energy, which would reduce the weight and increase the muscular effort and so 'toughness'.

Most farmed animals are fed specialized foods which accelerate growth, and antibiotics to reduce the dangers of infection, often caused by the diet and lifestyle. Animal exercise is deliberately kept to a minimum. Hormonal growth stimulators are added to the mix of artificial growth-enhancing foods. The result is that a modern carcass contains 25–30% fat. In contrast the fat content of free-living herbivores is usually under 4%.

A CALF'S LIFE

Even fifty years ago the raising of beef, for example, was very different from today. Cattle grazed freely in open fields, moving from pasture to pasture. When they were hungry they ate, and when they were not they slept.

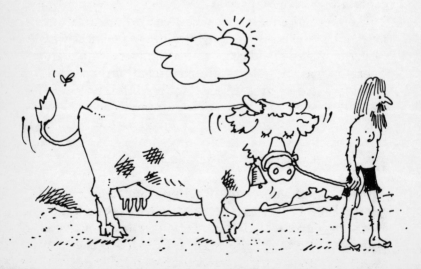

Animals grew strong, tended to be lean and were infinitely healthier than modern cattle. A calf reached maturity in two or three years.

Industrialized farming has reduced this period to around 18 months. Almost as soon as the calf is born it is placed on specialized feedstuffs, a mixture of milk powder, synthetic vitamins, minerals and antibiotics. This is largely in order to prevent any interruption of the mother cow's milk supply, which is saved for sale to consumers.

The calf is given special food and is allowed minimal exercise, which results in rapid weight gain. This food is eventually replaced by either pasture grass or, more commonly, processed food, premixed with antibiotics and other drugs to encourage further growth.

At the one-year stage, weighing some 230 kilos, the calf is usually placed in a pen, having been wormed and rid of parasites. There it remains for the rest of its life, fed around the clock, in a constantly lit environment. The food, which is frequently replenished, comprises high protein and high carbohydrate ingredients. It also contains urea carbohydrate and artificial fibre (often made of minced newspapers), with added molasses, plastic pellets and treated wood mixtures.

This is not a universal pattern, but is certainly the dominant method of producing meat in industrial farm units. And there are other techniques to increase weight. The use of the female hormone stilboestrol on young steers can produce a 10–15% weight increase with 10–15% less food for the animal. Heifers are fed other hormones, such as melengestrol acetate, which reduces their sex drive, alters the metabolism, and further increases weight gain. Tranquillizers are frequently used to cut down physical activity and increase the food intake.

To reduce the diseases resulting from this unnatural diet and lifestyle, additional antibiotics are added to the food. And in recent years, insecticide powders have been sprayed and dusted onto animals. Evidence that this is absorbed into their systems is found in the fact that the

manure they then produce becomes sterile (i.e. flies will
not lay their eggs in it).

Having gained a great deal of weight the animal is
finally sent for slaughter, after receiving additional
boosters of antibiotics.

THE MEAT WE EAT

The health implications of these practices is mind-
boggling. Rudolph Ballentyne MD points out that
animals raised in this fashion often develop cancers of
various sorts.[38] 'While these tumours are removed in the
slaughterhouse before the meat is marketed, it seems
clear that such animals cannot provide a high quality
of food.'

This is an understatement. Pigs are also frequently
fed in this manner, and some die of heart attacks on the
way to market.

HUMAN HEALTH IMPLICATIONS

The hormones used in animal husbandry have been
connected with various undesirable effects in humans,
including breast cancer, fibroid tumours, excessive
menstrual bleeding and impotence in men. Ballentyne
informs us that the incidence of vaginal cancer in the
daughters of women given stilboestrol is well
documented. What the effects of these hormones, which
remain present in meat, will be on the population over
a lengthy period, is unknown.

In the United States, inspectors examine slaughtered
livestock for gross defects, such as diseased organs,
tumours, bruising, abcessed livers and faecal
contamination. The inspection is brief and any cancer
found is cut out, the remainder of the carcass going on
to be processed.[39]

No current figures are available, but it is known that
in 1954, two and a half million cancerous carcasses were
consumed in the USA.

CHICKENS AND PIGS

Factory farmed chickens are often diseased. The chances of inspecting them adequately in the few seconds allocated is minimal, especially as the types of cancer present in many chickens are not visible to the naked eye. Outbreaks of leukemia and leucosis, forms of cancer which affect chickens in broiler houses, are increasing at an alarming rate.[40] Many birds die of cancer before they reach market, but the birds are so young when sent to the packing station that the disease has often not fully manifested itself. They are slaughtered and prepared for the oven by the million in this state of health.

Poultry is also fed with antibiotics and other drugs, in much the same manner as cows. Residues remain in the meat and these are eaten by the consumer.

It is much the same with pigs. Dense stocking rates increase efficiency and profitability; they also increase disease risk. 90% of our pigs suffer from some sort of clinical or subclinical disease.

Much of the meat that passes inspection is severely tainted with bacterial contamination. The chief of New Jersey's veterinary public health programme warned that no current method of meat or poultry inspection can assure disease-free raw meat or poultry products. Reliance on official inspection alone is likely to result in countless cases of food poisoning, such as salmonellosis and trichinosis.

And there are yet further concerns – the use of tenderizers (enzymes), preservatives and colouring factors in meat; and the additives in processed meats like pies and sausages, some of which have serious health implications.

COOKING METHODS

One of the commonest parasites in cattle, sheep and pigs is toxoplasma gondii. This requires a cooking period of not less than 20 minutes at a temperature of 80°C to destroy it.

Studies of current methods of preparation, especially in fast food restaurants, show that whether pan-fried meat balls, or pork chops, or even cooked spare ribs are considered, a high proportion fail to achieve either the temperature or the length of time required for safety.[41]

A further study examined the cooking of beef hamburgers and T-bone beef cuts over a hot plate. The maximum temperature in the centre of the hamburger during the average cooking time of five to ten minutes was 49°. With extended cooking, it could reach 60°, but any further cooking rendered the meat inedible. Steaks reached temperatures between 32°C and 35°C. This consistently failed to render the internal parasites harmless.

TOUGH BACTERIA

Bacteria which are constantly exposed to antibiotics eventually become resistant to them. The diseases which the bacteria produce are thus impervious to antibiotic treatment.

There has been a remarkable increase in the number and type of resistant bacteria in farm animals, including many strains of food-poisoning micro-organisms, such as salmonella. People who become poisoned by contaminated meat are therefore at greater risk, since treatment by antibiotics can often be ineffective.

The National Communicable Disease Centre in the USA estimates that about 38 million Americans suffer varying degrees of salmonella poisoning each year, mainly from contaminated meat. Avoiding such hazards either means not eating meat or ensuring its adequate cooking. Oven roasting is the surest method of achieving this.

FAT: THE FACTS

When considering fat, one more chemical danger becomes apparent. Many animals accumulate and store pesticide residues in their fat. The high level of fat in modern animals brings the risk that they will ingest excessive amounts of these chemicals, which remain in the body (stored in the liver or in fat deposits) for years. Again the long-term implications are not known.

The key difference between the fat of domesticated animals and that in free-living animals (game) is its composition. The fat found in game contains over five times the polyunsaturated fat found in livestock. Not only does the body of the farm-bred cow contain nearly 30% fat, but the type of fat is of the undesirable saturated variety.

Nearly 4% of the fat in wild animals is a most valuable substance known as EPA (eicosapentenoic acid). This is a long chain polyunsaturated fatty acid (PUFA for short). EPA is thought to be the prime reason for the healthy hearts of the Eskimos, as it protects against the build-up of atheromas in the blood vessels. EPA has been effective in the treatment of rheumatoid arthritis. The meat of farm animals contains barely a trace of EPA.

CHOLESTEROL CONTENT

There is little difference between the cholesterol content of the meat of free-living and domesticated animals, and the cholesterol intake in Paleolithic times was much the same as that of today, but without the harmful consequences.

The reason is that the amount of cholesterol found in the bloodstream has very little to do with the amount of cholesterol eaten. High cholesterol levels are linked to the quantities of saturated fats and sugars eaten, both of which played a much smaller part in Paleolithic diets than in modern diets. A further important anticholesterol factor in Paleolithic diets was the high fibre intake.

The ratio between the different kinds of fat in the diet is important in health terms, particularly that between polyunsaturated and saturated fats. The Senate Select Committee on Nutrition and Human Needs recommended that the ratio in modern diets should be increased to about 1.00 (equal amounts of saturated and polyunsaturated fats). In the United Kingdom the current ratio of 0.24 (four times more saturated fat than polyunsaturated) is frighteningly low.

Experience in the States has proved that changes in diet (and therefore of these ratios) can dramatically reduce the incidence of cardiovascular deaths. Although still in the midst of an epidemic of deaths from cardiovascular disease (coronaries, strokes, etc.), the USA has reversed a rising trend. The UK has not only failed to stem this rising tide of death and disablement, often of young people, but has shown a continuing increase in these conditions.

The cost in economic terms, and in terms of human waste and suffering, is enormous. In the USA alone some 250,000 people under the age of 50 are struck down each year by cardiovascular disease.

TOTAL FAT INTAKE

Cardiovascular diseases are absent in primitive man, and the ratio between polyunsaturated and saturated fats is a major reason why.

As a percentage of the diet overall, fats play a larger part in the USA than in the UK, providing 42% of the total energy intake. The Senate Committee has requested the US public to cut this down to 30%. In the UK 38% of energy intake is derived from fats of all sorts, and NACNE has also suggested that this be reduced to 30%.

Our Paleolithic ancestors, despite eating heroic quantities of meat, derived barely 21% of their energy from fats of all sorts.

MONOUNSATURATED OILS AND HEART HEALTH

The important monounsaturated fatty acids are almost totally absent in domesticated meats, but amount to almost a third of the fat contained in game.

Monounsaturated oils are also found in olive oil. In those countries where olive oil is a staple part of the diet, such as the Mediterranean countries of Greece, Italy, and Yugoslavia, cardiovascular disease is very uncommon.

A recent trial conducted at the University of Texas showed that monounsaturated oils, such as olive oil, are superior to polyunsaturated oils, such as safflower and sunflower oil, in reducing cholesterol levels in the blood. Monounsaturated oils are also better synthesized in the body.

These oils are also found abundantly in the Stone Age diet.

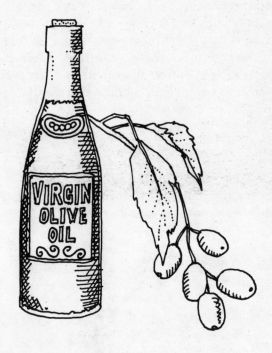

BOWEL PUTREFACTION

Meat-eaters face a potential problem in the length of human digestive systems. Relative to their size, carnivores have short bowels and vegetarian animals have long bowels. In this spectrum man fits into the vegetarian category. The length of the bowel affects the breakdown of foods after they have been eaten. Plant protein decays, and there are relatively few undesirable byproducts from this process. Meat and other animal proteins do not decay; they putrefy. Putrefaction is a process of breakdown which produces a number of toxic byproducts, and which is potentially dangerous to the body, unless the putrefying material is swiftly eliminated.

A Stone Age diet includes a high fibre content which ensures rapid bowel transit time (the time food takes to pass through and out of the digestive system). A modern Western diet causes a slow bowel transit time and putrefaction of the bowel contents can occur. This is thought to relate to bowel cancer, which is rare in vegetarians and unknown in primitive people. So anyone adopting the meat option should also ensure a high fibre intake, to ensure the full benefits of Paleolithic nutrition.

MEDIEVAL PEASANT DIET

The quality (or lack of it) of modern diet is put in perspective by comparison with that of country peasants in medieval Europe. Although obliged, under the feudal

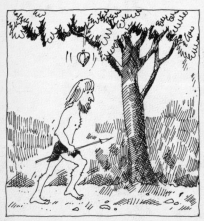
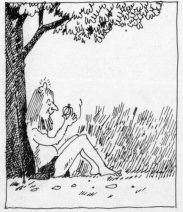

system, to perform a variety of duties for the landowner (such as ploughing and harvesting), they had livestock of their own and were permitted to grow some of their own crops. Their diet was far from meagre.

Three meals daily was the norm, which included bread, porridge, cheese, milk, seasonal vegetables and also dried vegetables (beans, etc.), fish and meat (either livestock or game).

Like hunter-gatherer people today, they ate the whole animal – liver, kidneys, lights (lungs) and all other offal, as well as muscle meat. Wild fruits and berries were present in the hedgerows, as were nuts, especially hazels. Country people were noted for their hunting and poaching talents, and wild life was plentiful.

Michael and Sheilagh Crawford have described the meats available.[42] 'There were deer in the woods, wild pigs, and birds of all types, from swans to starlings, were

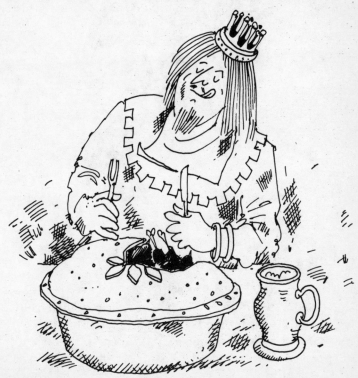

acceptable, and made succulent dishes. We are inclined
to leave to nursery rhymes the fact that the King must
be offered "four and twenty blackbirds baked in a pie".
We also tend to forget that even in our own century, the
local butchers did a good trade in quail, pheasant,
partridge, pigeon and wild duck; and until myxomatosis,
rabbits and hare were everyday dishes, and regularly
found on menus.'

In addition, a wide variety of seafood was available,
including a great many shellfish, and seaweed was often
eaten in many coastal areas. Wild birds' eggs were also
consumed.

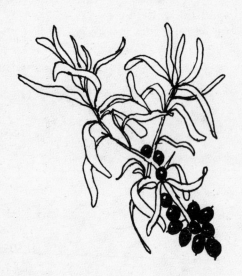

Sea buckthorn

AND TODAY?

In Europe today there are still areas where the eating
of game is common, particularly varieties of bird life. The
use of small birds for food is widespread in Mediterranean
countries. If meat is to be eaten, game should be sought.
Failing access to a reasonable supply of venison, hare,
wild birds and so on, then truly free-range fowl, such as

chicken and turkey, should be considered. There are many smallholders who supply such fare in country areas, and many butchers will stock seasonally available game, especially if demand increases.

In cities it can be more of a problem. London has a few butchers who will meet this need (Wholefood Butchers of Paddington Street is one). In the USA there are chains of health supermarkets, such as 'Mrs Gooch's Ranch Market' in California, who guarantee that their meat has been raised naturally, free of chemical and hormone additives.

A further option is fish, which remains relatively unspoiled. Fresh river or sea fish is a logical alternative for those who cannot obtain game or free-range fowl but want animal protein in their diet.

MARKET FORCES

The chances of everybody obtaining adequate supplies of game are not great. But were the meat production process to be altered, it might be possible to ensure lean farm-produced meat for the public, in place of game. Forage would replace cereals and protein additives, making ecological and economic sense, and allowing a better quality of life for the animal.

This could only occur as a result of consumer demand, with the consumer refusing to buy fatty meats and insisting on lean meat. The reduction of Europe's beef mountain would be a further result, since less actual weight of beef would reach the market.

There are some indications of change in farming practices. The *Sunday Times* recently reported (8 June 1986): 'Britain's farms are going to change. They haven't much choice – people are consuming less of their traditional products'. Their figures show market forces at work: in 1980 people in England and Wales consumed on average over 6½ kilos per year of pork; this dropped to only 5 kilos per head in 1985. Milk consumption fell too.

The article discusses a report by Reading University's

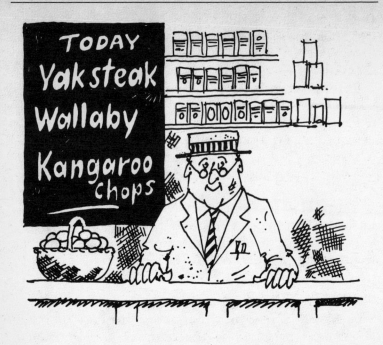

Centre for Agricultural Strategy, produced on behalf of the Ministry of Agriculture, which looks at the prospect of 2½ million acres being taken out of agriculture, over the next 10 years, as a result of the decrease in milk and lamb production. The report considers the practicalities of raising new meats, among them kangaroo, wallaby and yak, since their low fat content makes them more suitable to consumer requirements. These ideas may not yet have caught the farmer's or the public's imagination, but they do indicate general trends.

More likely, the report suggests, is an increase in free-range farming, especially of pigs and chicken. Free-range eggs have risen in popularity and, despite costing more than battery eggs, now account for 5% of the market, compared with 1% only five years ago.

Looking at the vegetarian trend, the report notes that 'if the UK were to change to vegetarianism, 90% of farmland would lie unused'. This is because less land is required to raise food for vegetarians. Animals eat huge amounts of grain and other plant products, to produce smaller quantities of food for people.

The market trend already seems to be away from traditional meat production towards a type of food which, without most consumers knowing it, accords with Stone Age standards.

4.
THE GREAT MILK DEBATE

The fact that two-thirds of the world's adult population is quite unable to digest milk, but is none the worse for it, should be borne in mind as we consider animal milk as a food.

With arguments ranging from 'milk is an essential human food' to the exact opposite, which insists that 'humans should not consume cow's milk', there are all the elements of an insoluble debate. On one hand we find the general claim that milk is a desirable and important part of the modern diet. This is countered by those who

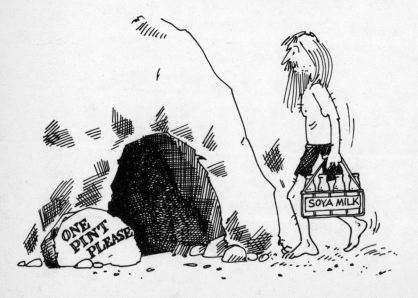

call it 'moo glue' and with unfeigned disgust suggest it should play no part at all in our dietary pattern.

Hardly any hunter-gatherer people consume milk, with the notable exception of the Masai, who drink it blended with fresh blood and appear to thrive on this mixture (supplemented with fruits, roots and berries). Paleolithic people drank no milk at all, apart from breast milk as infants.

Humans have been consuming milk for just 400 generations, too brief a time in genetic terms for our digestive apparatus to have become more than marginally adjusted to it. The enzyme lactase is required to digest milk sugar (lactose). Infants are designed to live on their mother's milk, and therefore have a reasonable supply of this enzyme. Most adults have little or no lactase.

MILK INTOLERANCE

Anyone with lactase deficiency who consumes milk will suffer from chronic or intermittent diarrhoea, bloating, flatulence or abdominal pain. Often the symptoms are mild, but sometimes they can require hospitalization.

The majority of people lose their lactase partly or totally when still young. The amount of residual lactase activity which remains in adult life determines the degree of symptoms that may occur when milk is consumed. Most adults retain sufficient lactase activity to be able to tolerate a small quantity of milk. Half a tumbler of milk will often be acceptable, whereas a large glass will produce symptoms.

It has been estimated that over 90% of the world's adult population is lactase deficient.[43] Looking at the differing racial responses to milk, the further north one travels in Europe, the better milk is generally tolerated. Oriental peoples seldom consume milk and many regard cheese with distaste.

Approximate percentage of adult lactase deficiency in different populations

Japan, China and Far East	100%
Africa (Negroid people)	100%
Africa (Hamite people)	10%
USA (blacks)	73%
USA (whites)	6–15%
USSR (Moscow area)	25%
England	25–30%
Greece	70–80%
Switzerland/Finland	17%
Sweden/Denmark	3%

The age at which lactase activity ceases is variable. The degree of lactase deficiency found in Australian aboriginals living a hunter-gatherer way of life show adults to be almost entirely lactase deficient, and most children unable to digest milk by the time they are six years old.[44] In Finland the decrease occurs between the ages of 10 and 20.

In Thailand the 'switch-off' is at age two. Even if milk feeding continues beyond this age, lactase production ceases. This indicates that the decrease in lactase activity is related to genetic control and is not simply a response to feeding patterns.

OVERCOMING LACTASE DEFICIENCY

Recognition of widespread lactase deficiency has led to suggestions designed to overcome it. One solution was suggested by the habits of the Masai. It is known that even if inadequate lactase is present in the gut, small amounts of milk can still be digested. This facility is increased if the milk is mixed with another form of food. Thus mixing milk with oil or sucrose makes it more digestible. The Masai mix it with whole blood, with similar results.

Another method which aids digestion of milk is to combine it with various bacterial cultures, which virtually predigest it. Sour milk, acidophilus milk and yoghurt are examples of this. When milk is taken in these forms, the body is largely spared the problem of breaking down the lactose, as this has been done by friendly bacteria.

A MUTANT EFFECT?

Arne Dahlqvist, a leading researcher, tells us:[45]

'Lactase persistence – ie. to keep the intestinal lactase activity throughout life – is a mutation. It can be speculated that we originally had (and most humans still have) a cut-off mechanism, that at a certain age decreases the production of intestinal lactase. This mechanism was damaged by mutation several thousand years ago. The mutant gene yielded a valuable ability to consume milk (in some people) throughout life, which considerably improved the nutrition, and made the owner "better fit for life".'

This 'advantage' is not universally appreciated, however. There are many indications of the undesirability of milk as a food in adult life and of cow's milk as a food for babies. Not being able to digest milk may be a distinct advantage, rather than the converse.

MILK HAZARDS

There is a proven link between milk consumption in populations with adult lactase (mainly Northern Europeans) and the presence of senile cataracts. Simoons describes this and maintains that milk consumption is a direct causative factor.[46] The more milk such a population consumes, as a whole, the higher is the incidence of cataracts.

Racial origins influence the effects of lactase deficiency. Coates has described a trial in which this was assessed:[47] 'Diarrhoea was caused by 50 grams of lactose in all 30 Chinese from Hong Kong, Malaysia and Singapore, in all 8 New Guinea natives, and all out of 4 Indians. Control subjects were Australian students of Caucasian (white) background, of whom none had diarrhoea. When 80 grams were tested, the subjects in the test had abdominal pain, bloating and occasional vomiting, and one of the control subjects had diarrhoea.' Coates pointed out that 'some Caucasoids are also allergic to cow's milk and to protein milk products such as cheese, which can be the cause of such complaints as ulcerative colitis, eczema and other allergies.'

MILK AND CALCIUM

One argument used in support of milk is that it provides calcium in good quantities. However, the research of Eaton and Konner indicates that, without any milk in their diets, the daily calcium intake of both Paleolithic people and modern hunter-gatherers is nearly 1600 mg.

By comparison, an average American diet today, with its high dairy product intake, provides 740 mg. The level suggested by the Senate Committee is between 800 and 1200 mg of calcium per day. Stone Age diets provide this, and more, without milk. Foods such as apples and cabbage offer very high calcium levels. If milk products are desired, those like yoghurt, with lactobacilli, are best, or soya milk for those with milk intolerance.

Sometimes, milk is recommended to correct a calcium deficiency, when in fact it will frequently have a deleterious effect. This applies particularly to middle-aged women in Western society suffering from demineralization of the bones (osteoporosis). Osteoporosis takes place when the bones lose their calcium, usually after the menopause. This results in many women suffering bone fractures after even slight injuries, because of the fragile bones. It is often accompanied by calcification of joints and circulatory vessels, and other associated health disturbances.

One standard piece of advice to women in this position is to consume more milk, as a source of calcium. However, a study, described in the *British Medical Journal* (18 January 1986), of women suffering from osteoporosis showed a high level of lactase deficiency. Their diets contained satisfactory amounts of calcium, but this came from milk sources, and because of their lactase intolerance, they were unable to absorb the calcium. Women who were not lactase intolerant, and who were consuming similar amounts of calcium in their diet, were not osteoporotic.

It was concluded that in the case of osteoporotic women who were lactase deficient, the advice to consume milk would have been of no benefit at all. Rather it would have added to their problems by causing the introduction of other, mainly digestive, symptoms.

THE SQUATTERS WITHIN

The symptoms of lactose intolerance are caused by the activity of bacteria, which thrive on the unabsorbed lactose in the digestive tract.

Paradoxically, these symptoms can occur in people who have adequate lactase and do not always occur in people who are lactase deficient. The reason is the vast difference which exists in the bacterial flora of different people, which relates very much to the individual's overall dietary pattern.

When we eat we are feeding not only ourselves but a veritable army of squatters, who live in our digestive tracts. Some 100 different species of micro-organisms and fungi inhabit each one of us. Most are benign and even useful. Some, however, are potentially harmful, and a poor diet can create imbalances which allow the less friendly bacteria to dominate.

The use of fermented cultures such as yoghurt, which contains live bacteria, are useful in repopulating the digestive tract with friendly bacteria.

MILK TREATMENT

Most milk sold today is pasteurized in an attempt to protect the health of the public. This process requires that milk be heated to either 62°C for 30 minutes or 72°C for 15 minutes. As a result some, but not all, bacteria present are destroyed.

All proteins are made of amino acids, and their relationships with each other can be altered by heat. During pasteurization, weak linking bonds may be strengthened. This can result in a degree of coagulation or clumping of molecules, when they eventually come into contact with the acids of the digestive system.

If, on the other hand, untreated milk is brought quickly to the boil, this strengthening of weak bonds does not happen. Rather, the process actually causes the weak protein bonds to weaken further, making the milk more digestible.

Therefore if milk is consumed, raw unpasteurized milk should be chosen. This is available in some farm shops and health food shops. Boiled milk is more easily digested than pasteurized or homogenized milk, even by those with plentiful lactase.

IS MILK A HUMAN FOOD?

Human milk is designed for humans, cows' milk for baby cows. There is a difference between them, cows' milk being some 400% higher in protein content. This difference relates very closely to the maturing process in the respective intended (by nature) recipients. Cows have a remarkable growth rate, increasing in size and weight in a short space of time, to reach maturity. Humans take far longer to mature, as do all primates.

Milk is nature's food to newborn animals. Depending on the time required for them to mature, the drinking of mother's milk lasts an appropriate length of time. Humans require the longest of all to reach adulthood, and the lactating period is proportionally higher. The digestive organs of human babies are programmed to receive milk until the development of teeth makes the eating of solid food both possible and desirable. At this stage weaning should commence, and milk from the mother should gradually be stopped.

There is no physiological reason for adult humans to consume milk of any sort. And for most people this is confirmed by their inability to digest it. No other animal on earth receives milk after it is weaned.   *cats*

ALLERGIES

There has in recent years been a surge of investigation into the widespread problems associated with allergy. Many doctors who have concentrated their research into the environmental and dietary factors involved (clinical ecologists) advocate a Stone Age diet for their patients.

This automatically removes all dairy produce and processed food. In many cases this is all that is required to recover good health. Milk appears to be the single most potent allergy-causing agent. Asthma, eczema, skin rashes, chronic nasal and sinus problems, tonsilitis, bowel irregularity, hyperactivity, depression, forms of arthritis, and migraines have all been shown to be caused by milk intolerance.

SYMPTOMS OF ALLERGY

Allergy may be implicated if any of the following symptoms are noted:

- Persistent fatigue which is not improved by rest.
- Problems associated with weight – either persistent over- or under-weight, or marked fluctuations in weight.
- Unexplained swellings on the face, hands, abdomen or ankles.
- Palpitations, especially after meals.
- Unexplained and excessive sweating, unrelated to exercise.

These and many other symptoms are caused by milk intolerance, and advice should be sought from a doctor who specializes in nutritional methods of treatment, if in any doubt.

Milk is one of the major changes we have had thrust upon our bodies in the past few thousand years. We have not adapted to it very well. The dairy industry is a human creation, and the animals involved certainly do not benefit from being turned into virtual milk machines, requiring constant medication to maintain a state of perpetual lactation. The relative differences which exist between goats', sheep's and cows' milk are of little relevance to the overall argument. Some milks are more easily coped with than others but all are designed for the offspring of their species – not for humans.

CHILDREN AND MILK

Children are well provided with lactase for digestion of their mother's milk, so can they not cope equally well with cows', goats' or sheep's milk? In answer to this, the prestigious medical journal *Paediatrics* specifically advised that whole cows' milk should not be fed to infants during the first year of life.[48] Infants fed on whole cows' milk are prone to occult gastro-intestinal bleeding, iron deficiency and allergic reactions. Furthermore, the health hazards of lactose intolerance – milk-born infections and high serum cholesterol levels (associated with heart disease) – remain as problems in the post-infancy period.

Australian trials have found a link between hyperactivity in children and milk consumption. It was found that the stool samples of hyperactive children contained high levels of tyrosine, an amino acid found in milk. Tyrosine excess had previously been implicated in behavioural disorders, and it was concluded that a combination of a high carbohydrate diet (mainly sugar) and milk caused the hyperactivity, since carbohydrate minimizes the absorption of other amino acids which compete with tyrosine. Tyrosine evolves biochemically into elements which affect brain function. Sugar and milk together in the diet cause the brain literally to become over stimulated and hyperactivity follows. Our Paleolithic ancestors had no such problems.

The use of milk clearly presents a number of health hazards to infants and children, as well as to adults.

5.
VITAMIN C

Vitamin C is one of the most important of all nutrients. Its deficiency in humans relates directly to a range of symptoms, most notably immune deficiency and lowering of the body's defence mechanisms.

The differences between the intake achieved by a modern diet, that suggested by experts as desirable, and the amount consumed on a Stone Age diet, are dramatic. The inferior health of modern industrialized societies, compared to the Stone Age, is thought by many to be largely related to this disparity in vitamin C intake. Why and how this has happened is a fascinating example of genetic change, which subsequently proved to be undesirable.

THEN AND NOW

Most Westerners today have an average daily consumption of under 80 mg of vitamin C. The recommended daily allowance (RDA) which health authorities say we need for health is between 40 and 60 mg daily. The Paleolithic diet, according to Eaton and Konner, provided around 400 mg of vitamin C daily.[49] Modern hunter-gatherer intake is about the same. In making these estimates some fruits commonly eaten by particular tribes have been ignored, as they might have distorted the findings. Many are eaten infrequently, but their content of vitamin C is phenomenal. The Australian wild green plum for example contains 315 mg of vitamin C per 100 grams.

Many tribes on different continents, including the San, Hadza, Kung, Kade, Tasady and Aboriginals, were studied by Eaton and Konner. They reached the conclusion that 'the vitamin intake of Paleolithic human beings would have substantially exceeded ours, irrespective of the amount of meet in the diet.' Since marginal, and sometimes clinical, nutrient deficiency can be demonstrated in many strata of affluent societies today, this is of some significance.

THE IMPORTANCE OF VITAMIN C

Some vital substances are manufactured within the body, from raw material provided in the diet. Protein, for example, is made up of about 20 components called amino acids. Most of these can be made in the body from other substances. However there are eight amino acids which adults have to provide through their diet before the body is able to make protein. Because we cannot manufacture these eight amino acids, they are called 'essential amino acids'. There are other amino acids which become essential at particular times of life, such as childhood, and these are called 'contingent amino acids'.

Vitamin C plays a key role in forming collagen, which is vital for the growth and repair of body tissues, gums, blood vessels, teeth and bones. Vitamin C is important in the absorption of iron into the body. It prevents viral and bacterial infections, helps decrease blood cholesterol, aids in healing wounds, is a natural laxative, reduces the chances of bloodclots forming, slows down the ageing process and, being an anti-oxidant, detoxifies certain undesirable elements in the body. Vitamin C reduces the chances of allergic symptoms developing and plays a major anti-cancer role.

Somewhere in evolutionary prehistory, humans lost the ability to manufacture vitamin C for themselves. It became an essential nutrient.

EVOLUTIONARY ADVANTAGE?

In evolutionary terms it is an advantage for any animal to shed the burden of having to manufacture a substance for itself, if that substance is freely available in the diet. Linus Pauling explains this in the following passage:[50]

'Consider the epoch, early in the history of life on earth, when the early animals of the species nourished themselves by eating plants, possibly together with other food. All plants contain thiamine. Accordingly the animals would have in their bodies thiamine that they had ingested, as well as thiamine that they had synthesized, by use of their own synthesizing mechanisms. Now, let us assume that a mutant animal appeared in the population, an animal that, as the result of the impact of a cosmic ray on a gene, or the action of some other mutagenic agent, had lost the biochemical machinery that still permitted the other members of the species to manufacture thiamine from other substances. The amount of thiamine provided by the ingestion of food would suffice to keep the mutant animal well nourished, essentially as well nourished as the unmutated animals, and the mutant would have the advantage over the unmutated animals, in that it would be liberated from the burden of the machinery for manufacturing its own thiamine. As a result the mutant would have more offspring than the other animals of the population. By reproduction the mutated animal would pass its advantageously mutated genes along to some of its offspring, and they too would have more than the average number of offspring. Thus in the course of time this advantage, the advantage of not having to do the work of manufacturing thiamine, or to carry within itself the machinery for this manufacture, could permit the mutant type to replace the original type.'

Of course, had such a mutation occurred, and the nutrient (be it thiamine or another) not been readily available in the food, the mutation would not have been an advantage. The genetic pattern would have died out, because the mutant animal would not have reproduced adequately. The 'normal', unmutated animals would have continued to reproduce and would have overridden the mutant gene.

EXPERIMENTAL PROOF

Research using bacterial strains with very short reproductive cycles allows alterations in genetic pattern to be studied in ways which would be difficult in large creatures, where the timescale of observing successive generations makes such study difficult or impossible.

These experiments show clearly that the burden of using the machinery to synthesize a nutrient is a major disadvantage, when one strain is in competition with another which has lost the need for such machinery. Those bacteria which still have laboriously to manufacture the nutrient lose out, in evolutionary terms, and die out.

The number of generations required, starting with equal numbers of bacterial cells, to reach the point where the 'victorious' strain has one million times as many cells as the unmutated groups, is around fifty. For humans this would mean 1,000 to 1,500 years, taking 20 years as a generation. This assumes that humans are sufficiently closely interconnected for genetic change to be passed around through intermarriage. Since this is not the case, and humans are not cells in a culture dish, we can only take the broad gist of these experiments.

However, if we go back far enough in time, when humans were confined to a small number living in a limited region of the earth, such genetic change could well be acquired by the entire race over a period of several hundred thousand years. Just such a change has occurred in relation to vitamin C.

OTHER VITAMINS

Like most animals we require a set of basic nutrients in our food in order to survive. These include vitamin A, which all vertebrate animals need for functions like skin health, normal bone development and visual function. We also require the B group of vitamins as we cannot manufacture them in the body in any significant quantity, as do some other animals, such as the pig, rat, cat and cow.

Since humans and these animal groups have all lost the ability to synthesize these nutrients, mutation must have taken place very early in the earth's history. Some ancient ancestor, common to both humans and these animals, and with these nutrients available in its food, must have mutated (as in the thiamine example) and gained an evolutionary advantage by losing the need to manufacture vitamins A and B.

VITAMIN C AND ANIMALS

Vitamin C synthesis has been retained by most animals. Humans and the other primates, however, all require vitamin C in their diets. The loss of the ability to make vitamin C must have occurred in a common ancestor, shared by humans and the primates. This probably took place some 25 million years ago, according to Pauling.

A few other animals, such as the guinea pig, the Indian fruit-eating bat, and one or two birds, also require vitamin C from their diets. Their mutations were probably independent of those which affected the primates and humans, being useful for them, and connected with their ample access to foods rich in ascorbic acid.

But why have similar mutations relating to vitamin C not also occurred in other animals, such as cows, chickens and horses, who have been genetically relieved of the task of making their own vitamins A and B?

According to Linus Pauling, 'the fact that most species have not lost the ability to manufacture their own ascorbic acid shows that the supplies of ascorbic acid available generally in foodstuffs are not sufficient to provide optimum amounts of this substance. Only in an unusual environment, in which the available food provided an unusually large amount of ascorbic acid, have circumstances permitted a species of animal to abandon its own powers of synthesis of this important substance.'[51]

These very changes were allowed in the early humans or their immediate predecessors because there were then unusually large amounts of vitamin C available to them, since they were living in primeval jungles on a diet of fruits, berries and vegetables.

A DISADVANTAGEOUS ADVANTAGE?

The modern survivors of the primates, such as the mountain gorilla, eat mainly fresh vegetation and their daily intake of vitamin C is around 4,500 mg. It is no wonder that evolution genetically allowed these great apes to stop producing vitamin C.

But the advantage for humans was put in question when the climatic changes of prehistory threw them out in to the scrub of Africa, to scrabble for their food. The chance of regaining a lost genetic trait is minimal, and in any case has not happened. Humans are dependent on a dietary source of vitamin C.

One accommodation we have made in response to this, however, is that our bodies have evidently learned to function on less vitamin C than previously.

VITAMIN C RECYCLED

Pauling argues that 'it is almost certain that some evolutionary effective mutations have occurred in man and his immediate predecessors rather recently (within the last two million years) such as to permit life to continue on an intake of ascorbic acid less than that provided by high-ascorbic-acid, raw plant foods. These mutations might involve an increased ability of the kidney tubules to pump ascorbic acid back into the blood from the glomerular filtrate (dilute urine, being concentrated for passage along the tubules) and an increased ability of certain cells to extract ascorbic acid from the blood plasma.'[52]

Organs such as the adrenal glands may act as a storehouse for vitamin C, releasing it when needed. Stress depletes adrenal supplies of vitamin C which is one reason why vitamin C is required in greater quantities in times of stress.

SCURVY

There is a large gap between the optimum level of nutrient intake at which *all* the needs of an animal, or human are met, and that at which obvious deficiency symptoms become apparent. Below a certain level of vitamin C consumption, the symptoms of scurvy will become manifest.

Scurvy is characterized by multiple haemorrhages. In adults, it is preceded by lassitude, weakness, irritability, vague muscle and joint pains and loss of weight. The earliest objective signs include bleeding gums, gingivitis and loosening of the teeth. Next come minute haemorrhages under the skin, followed by larger haemorrhages, often in the muscles, eyes or brain. There may be frequent bleeding from the nose, or bowel or bladder haemorrhages.

With slightly more vitamin C the body is just able to cope, but at a severely handicapped level of function. Intake over this level leads to what might be called 'average' health, the common norm in modern society, which in fact lies somewhere between rank deficiency and high level health.

ARE WE GETTING ENOUGH?

Optimum levels of any nutrient, including vitamin C, vary from person to person. Roger Williams refers us to an account in which one member of a crew of sailors is described as suffering from severe scurvy and as being at death's door while the others, subsisting on the same imperfect diet, are free of deficiency symptoms.

There is, according to Williams, 'a wide spread between the amount of vitamin C needed to prevent frank scurvy, and that required for the maintenance of best health. In young growing guinea pigs about 0.5 mg of ascorbic acid per day will protect against scurvy symptoms, but there are distinct gains in health when the intakes are up to 10 times this amount.'[53]

Studying the levels of vitamin C in the tissues of healthy volunteers, Williams found that in groups of as few as nine or ten individuals, vitamin C requirement differed by up to 400% to maintain healthy tissues. There is really no firm 'norm' for vitamin C intake.

Linus Pauling studied the amounts of various vitamins in over 100 raw, natural plant foods and calculated how much such food would be required to provide an average adult with a daily energy intake of 2,500 calories.[54] On a diet high in raw plant foods, most vitamins would be supplied at roughly three times the daily recommended allowance (RDA). In particular such a diet would provide fully 2,250 mg of vitamin C daily, some fifty times the official recommendation of 40–60 mg.

The hunter-gatherer of today consumes at least ten times the daily RDA amount of vitamin C, and probably more. The RDA of vitamin C provides enough to prevent widespread scurvy, and little more than that.

With Williams' work showing a range of requirements varying by 400% even in small groups, the real need of the population at large clearly cannot be met by sticking to the RDA guidelines. The RDA seems even more dubious if we consider the amount of vitamin C manufactured by animals which have not lost this facility. Irwin Stone reports that the rat synthesizes vitamin C at a rate of between 26 and 58 mg per kilogram of body weight.[55] For a human of 70 kilos (11 stone) that would mean 1,800 to 4,000 mg daily.

If the vitamin C manufactured by goats, cows, sheep and dogs is similarly extrapolated, the human requirement would approach 10,000 mg (10 grams) per day.

'It is hard', Pauling concludes, 'to believe that these animals would make this large amount of ascorbic acid if it were not beneficial to them, and also hard to believe that humans are so much different from other animals that they can keep in the best health with only two-hundredths of the amount they use.'

Coming closer to our own needs are those of various monkey species, medical research indicates that these animals, when maintained in laboratories in the best of health, require between 1,750 and 3,500 mg of vitamin C daily. Guinea pigs, which like humans have lost the ability to manufacture vitamin C, require an amount equivalent to 3,500 mgs. Since the average human diet has an intake of vitamin C of less than 100 mg daily, the implications of all this in health terms are enormous.

FOLK TRADITION

Ballentyne tells us that until recently, a wild plant common in North America known as boneset (*Eupatorium perfolatum*) was a favourite remedy in country areas.[56] Dried leaves were kept handy, and a bitter-tasting tea was made whenever illness threatened, often stopping it in its tracks, according to tradition. Analysis shows that the vitamin C content of the two or three cups usually consumed at such times would deliver between 10 and 30 grams of vitamin C – a truly enormous dose.

In India similar folk tradition calls for the preparation of a sour liquid made from a fruit known locally as amla. Only the size of a walnut, this fruit contains more than 10 times the vitamin C of an orange.

These are but two examples of the common use of vitamin C in folk tradition. It has protected generations

90

from deficiency. City dwelling has deprived many of us of such methods, necessitating supplemental forms of vitamin C from health food stores or pharmacies. Attention to diet could avoid this need.

WHO IS DEFICIENT?

Dr Emmanual Cheraskin, Emeritus Professor of Nutrition at Alabama University, tested large groups comprising people of different ages and social status, and found widespread vitamin C deficiency.[57]

Basu and Schorah defined two main divisions of vitamin C deficiency, the first showing what they term 'suboptimal' levels, the second showing frank scurvy symptoms.[58]

Percentage of individuals showing vitamin C deficiency in different social groups

GROUP	SUBOPTIMAL LEVELS OF VITAMIN C	WITH SCURVY
Young healthy	3%	0%
Elderly healthy	20%	3%
Elderly outpatients	68%	20%
Cancer patients	76%	46%
Institutionalized elderly	95%	50%
Institutionalized young	100%	30%

The truly frightening figures are those for people in institutions, such as hospitals, prisons and mental homes. There, almost all people, young or old, are deficient in vitamin C, and between a third and a half are suffering from real scurvy.

THE STONE AGE CONNECTION

Dr Cheraskin was fascinated by the research of Eaton and Konner into Paleolithic diet, and especially by their assessment of the Paleolithic vitamin C intake (around 400 mg daily).

On the hypothesis that relatively healthy people, free of symptoms are likely to have a vitamin C intake closer to the ideal than those who are unhealthy, Cheraskin evaluated the intake of over 1,000 doctors and their wives, who completed detailed food questionnaires to ascertain vitamin C consumption. They also answered a 'self-assessment' questionnaire on symptoms. Developed by the Cornell University Medical College, New York, the questionnaire has some 200 questions which are answered 'Yes' or 'No', and which establish the number of symptoms experience – from headaches to runny nose, constipation to depression.

Cheraskin found that the average daily vitamin C intake of the entire group was 327 mg, with some taking in only 15 mg per day and others over 1000 mg. Overall there was an average of 16 symptoms, with some people having none at all, and others as many as 125.

He then eliminated from the calculations all those with more than 30 symptoms. In this reduced group, vitamin C intake rose to average 335 mg per day. Removing those with more than 15 symptoms, average intake of vitamin C was up to 349 mg per day. By continually refining the remaining group until he reached the healthiest – those who had no symptoms at all – he found that the average intake of vitamin C rose correspondingly.

The more vitamin C, the fewer symptoms in the group. Those who had no symptoms averaged 410 mg per day of vitamin C – an amount almost identical to that found by Eaton and Konner to be the Paleolithic average intake.

VITAMIN C DEFICIENCY SYMPTOMS

These include:

- A tendency to haemorrhage internally, under the skin or in the joints (bruising easily is an early sign)

- Childhood rheumatic conditions
- Osteomyalitis (bone inflammation); fragility of bone
- Poor wound healing
- Gingivitis and dental disease (bleeding gums are an early sign)
- Gastrointestinal disorders (including lack of hydrochloric acid for digestion)
- Increased susceptibility to infection
- A tendency to spontaneous abortion and infertility
- Increased cholesterol in the blood (and so high risk of cardiovascular disease)
- Increased tendency to allergy
- Increased tendency towards cancer
- Increased incidence of sudden infant death syndrome (SIDS)
- Anaemia
- Cataracts
- Hormonal disorders

VITAMIN C SOURCES

Stone Age humans had a wide choice of fruits, berries and green plants readily available. A major part of any dietary pattern, be it meat-containing or vegetarian, should include a substantial number of these. It is particularly suggested that wild (free-growing) vegetables such as dandelions, comfrey and mustard greens, which are delicious as well as nutritious, be included in the diet. Methods of preparation are given in the recipe section.

Pauling's research classified fruits and vegetables into low C, intermediate C, high C and very high C groups:

Low C foods
apples, apricots, avocadoes, bananas, cherries, coconut, dates, figs, grapefruit, grapes, mangoes, nectarines, peaches, pears, pineapples, plums, crabapples, honeydew melon, watermelon
blackberries, blueberries, cranberries, raspberries,

redcurrants, gooseberries
beans, peas, bamboo shoots, carrots, celeriac root, celery,
cucumber, garlic, cloves, lettuce, okra, parsnips, potato,
pumpkin, onion, sweetpotato, yams

Intermediate C foods
oranges, lemons, limes, cantaloupe melon, ripe tomatoes,
strawberries
artichokes, asparagus, beet greens, chicory, Chinese
cabbage (Chinese leaves), fennel, radishes, spinach,
zucchini (courgettes), Swiss chard

High C foods
Brussels sprouts, cabbage, cauliflower, chives, collards,
mustard greens

Very high C foods
blackcurrants
broccoli spears, kale, parsley, hot chilli (green or red),
sweet peppers (green or red)

The low C list may come as a surprise. Its complement
of fruits, berries and vegetables are not, however, to be
disparaged, because they contain many valuable
materials, as well as their modest amounts of
vitamin C.

Those foods on the high and very high C lists should
be eaten as often as possible, and the more that is eaten
raw, the better.

COOKING: FOR BETTER OR WORSE?

Cooking has two somewhat contradictory effects on
vegetables. The heat breaks down the fibrous material
which locks many nutrients away from easy digestion
– so more vitamin A is derived from cooked carrots than
from raw ones. However heat also destroys some
nutrients, notably vitamin C.

A certain amount of cooking is desirable, but this
should be kept to a minimum, while still allowing the

breakdown of plant fibre. Stir-frying with little or no oil, steaming or very lightly boiling are recommended methods. The levels of vitamin C in high and very high C foods, of which our Stone Age ancestors ate liberally, are particularly reduced by long periods of cooking.

If such a high intake pattern is followed, supplementation is unnecessary. If a good supply of raw, fresh food is not eaten, however, a vitamin C supplement of between 400 and 800 mg daily is recommended, depending on stress levels and exposure to pollution. Both of these increase the body's requirement for vitamin C.

6.
COOKING, FLAVOURING AND CHEWING

Some foods are better digested when cooked, more easily yielding their nutrient store. The breakdown of the fibrous structure of vegetables, when exposed to heat, releases tightly bound substances for the digestive processes to work on. The heat expands the starch in the plant cells, rupturing the cellular walls. Similarly when meat is cooked the tough connective tissue is weakened and made more tender, so that nutrients are more easily derived.

Nevertheless there is some nutrient loss in any heating process from the destruction of vitamins and enzymes. Also, essential minerals are easily discarded in the cooking water. Once cells are weakened by cooking, oxidation of the exposed substances brings further nutrient loss if the food is not eaten immediately.

FIRE

Humans have used fire for hundreds of thousands of years. Whether it was used for cooking from the outset is a matter of debate, and there are few direct clues.

In prehistoric sites, some hearths excavated were built directly onto the ground, others on a stone base often hollowed out specifically for the purpose. Sometimes there was a covering of gravel, perhaps used as a means of

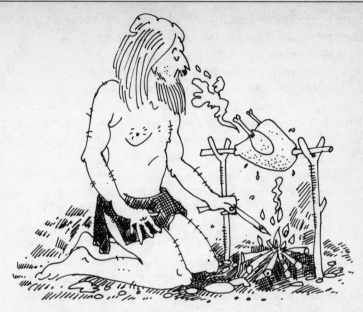

storing heat, others appear to be ovens. Wood or bone was the fuel, and the evidence suggests that meat was roasted or grilled and sometimes smoked over a green wood fire.

The first known practical use of fire was during the periods of glaciation, some 400,000 years ago. Evidence for this has been discovered in France, Italy, Hungary, Spain and China. Use of fire in Africa appears to have begun later, perhaps because of the warmer climate, or it may be that evidence has simply not yet come to light.

It is thought that the first fires used by early humans were lit from natually occurring fires and the use of flints for starting fire was a later accidental discovery.

COOKING: AN ECHO OF THE PAST?

Desmond Morris believes that we hearken back to our past when we cook food:[59]

'There are three alternative explanations. One is that it helps to simulate "prey" temperature. Although we no

97

longer consume freshly killed meat, we nevertheless devour it at much the same temperature as other carnivore species. Their food is hot because it has not yet cooled down: ours is hot because we have heated it.

Another interpretation is that we have such week teeth that we are forced to tenderize the meat by cooking it. But this does not explain why we should want to eat it while it is still hot, or why we should heat up many kinds of food that do not require tenderizing.

'The third explanation is that by increasing the temperature of the food we improve its flavour.'

In Morris' opinion, the heating and spicing of food relates not to our adopted pattern of meat-eating, but to our earlier primate past. The diet of a typical primate has a much wider variety of flavours than that of a carnivore. So by heating and spicing our foods, we reflect the subtle and varied flavours enjoyed by our early primate ancestors.

THE WAY WE EAT

Morris also points out that we differ from the primates by not continually eating. Rather, we lean towards the pattern of carnivores, who eat large meals, well spaced out.

The primate tendency to be continually munching certainly appears to exist for many people who constantly eat snacks. This behaviour is closer to our roots than that of those who gorge, like the great cats of Africa.

Fastidiousness, a liking for tasty variations in our eating, and the use of spices and flavour are all, according to Morris, signs of our early arborial origins. On the other hand, the desire to warm our food is possibly an echo of the memory of the heat of freshly killed meat, deriving from our period in the wilderness after vegetarianism was abandoned.

TO COOK OR NOT TO COOK?

Experiments indicate that, nutritionally, raw meat is far more desirable than cooked meat. This ignores the question of parasites and bacterial contamination already discussed.

Much of the meat consumed by hunter-gatherers is eaten raw.[60] This is true of the Eskimos, who eat raw blubber, liver, seal meat and fish. It is also true of numerous tribes who eat at least some meat and fish practically raw.

The late F. M. Pottenger MD carried out a series of classic experiments in the 1940s on the long-term effects of cooking protein foods. These convinced him that animals which live on protein, such as rats and cats, should eat at least two thirds of their food uncooked. He proved that cats raised on a diet of food one third raw and two thirds cooked could not normally survive and reproduce beyond the fourth month of their third generation. *in the wild?*

Within six months, cats eating predominantly cooked foods became ill. Incidence of allergy rose from 5% to 95%. All animals in the third generation suffered from chronic diseases, and from many acute infections which affect humans, including arthritis, dermatitis, gut disease, pneumonia, kidney disease and from allergies. They became more subject to infestation and intestinal parasites, and there was increasing incidence of vicious behaviour and homosexuality.

On the other hand, the cats on a diet two thirds raw and one third cooked reproduced indefinitely, with offspring that maintained good health all their lives, which were of normal length.

When cats in a degenerated state of health were given a diet of mainly raw food, it took between three and four generations to restore normal cat physiology and function.

Obviously, the sort of studies made by Pottenger on cats cannot be undertaken on humans. Still, they closely recall the findings of Weston Price in his detailed work on primitive peoples and their anatomy and dental health.[61]

Price travelled the world studying 14 different groups of people, most of whom followed a Stone Age way of life and eating pattern. He also made comparative studies of people from the same groups who had abandoned traditional eating for 'civilized' patterns. He produced copious photographic and other evidence, showing the pathetic degeneration in dental health resulting from a change to modern food and the rise of the diseases of civilization, previously unknown in these peoples.

DIETS ANCIENT AND MODERN

Price found that the children of adults who had adopted a modern diet had narrowed facial bones and dental arches, crowded teeth and dental decay. Genetically acquired defects such as cleft palate and clubfoot, previously unknown in these people, were first noted in such offspring. If tribal people who had conceived children after adopting civilized eating habits later returned to their tribal diets and again conceived, these children had marvellous wide faces and dental arches, with teeth free of decay.

This was an example of degeneration caused solely by nutritional manipulation which was not mediated by genetic factors and was reversible – but only in the first generation. Thereafter, as with Pottenger's cats, restoring normal physiology could be expected to take several generations.

Dr Price noted that 'almost all primitive diets studied contained at least four times the minimum requirements of nutrients, whereas the displacing nutrition of commerce, consisting largely of refined flour products, sugar, polished rice, jams, canned foods and vegetable fats has invariably failed to produce the minimum requirements.'

The results of a diet impoverished by processing and

overcooking are elaborated by Sir Robert McCarrison, who contrasted the health and physiques of people living on different diets in the Indian subcontinent.[62]

Some of the finest examples were the Mahratta, Sikhs and Pathans, who usually ate very high protein diets, as did the Tibetan hillmen, who were found to consume 6,000 calories of food daily, 175 grams of it from animal sources. By contrast Hunza tribesmen ate a mainly vegetarian diet, much of it raw. They had prime health and physiques and were very long lived.

Bengali and Madrasi people however, on an ill-constituted diet with little or no animal protein and rice as the major element, were poor physical specimens, in uncertain health.

Such studies demonstrate the importance of a balanced diet, the need for raw food to be a part of it, and how ill-health thrives on refined, excessively cooked and denatured foods.

HIGH NUTRIENT LEVELS

In the primitive tribes whose diets most closely resemble the Paleolithic one, we find that the minimum requirements for essential nutrients are exceeded by as much as 25 times, as in the case of magnesium. The soluble fat vitamins, such as A, E and K, are found in such diets at ten times the level thought adequate in our society. There are between two and eight times the minimum required levels of calcium, phosphorus and all water soluble nutrients (such as vitamins C and B) in these diets.

If we cook our food excessively, or eat refined processed food, a progressive deterioration like those found by Pottenger and Price will affect succeeding generations. Reversal of this process takes a long time and can only begin with the willing adoption, by us, of a reduction in 'civilized' foods. These should be replaced by as much unrefined, uncooked, whole food as is available. Approximately one third of this should be cooked and the remainder raw.

This may not always be easy, but if abundant fruit and salad accompanies those foods we find impossible to eat raw, giant strides will be made in the right direction.

IMPLICATIONS OF CHEWING

At the dawn of human existence all food was eaten uncooked plucked raw from the trees. Today, conditions preclude such a life for most of us and there are sound hygienic reasons for cooking in modern societies, where contamination from bacteria and parasites can be widespread.

A return to a basically raw food diet would require revolutionary changes in the time spent eating. Raw food takes longer to chew than cooked food. More frequent small meals might be necessary, as was the case when our primitive ancestors were still vegetarians.

Some anthropologists suggest that cooking has been a critical factor in human development. The shorter chewing time has allowed for a reduction in skull size, so that the heavy jaw and brow of the Neanderthal, which supported huge chewing muscles, have been replaced by a smaller bone structure.

The refashioning of the face has permitted more subtle speech, and has freed the face to be capable of intricate communication skills. Just as our ancestors freed their hands when they adopted the upright position, so they freed their faces by reducing the need for endless munching of raw food.[63]

With hands and face freed and with the development of skills and intelligence, the brain has grown, resulting in humanity's supremely gifted cerebral development. This is an appealing argument, although it must remain pure conjecture.

SENSIBLE COOKING

We are unlikely to return completely to raw food eating, though a majority of food should ideally be eaten raw.

Methods of cooking should destroy as little as possible of the food value. Those used traditionally in China are a good model. Wok frying (stir frying) uses the minimum of oil and is done by constant stirring and agitation of the food, so that heat causes the desirable breakdown of the food's tough internal structures, tenderizing it and making digestion and chewing easier, without undue nutrient loss.

Steaming also achieves this by heating the food without boiling away excessive amounts of nutrients. Baking has similar results.

A SWEET LEGACY?

Morris points out that a 'sweet tooth' is a primate characteristic, not found in carnivores.[64] 'As the natural food of primates becomes riper and more suitable for consumption, it usually becomes sweeter, and monkeys and apes have a strong reaction to anything which is strongly endowed with this taste.'

We too have a great difficulty in resisting sweet substances. Meals usually end with a sweet course and snacks are frequently sweet-tasting as, according to Morris, we revert to our primate 'scatter eating' pattern. The almost instinctive drive for sweet foods overrides our other instinctual reaction to food, its nutritive value. In a natural setting the two factors go hand in hand. As fruits ripen, they become both sweeter and more nutritive. Palatability is nutritious, in nature.

However, artificially sweetened foods have deprived us of the key nutrients, instead feeding us vast amounts of empty calories. These foods have little or no nutritive value, and often actually carry a negative impact, since they use up existing nutrients already present in the body. They have dominated Western eating in the latter part of the 20th century, where too much is eaten and too little value derived, so that obesity and disease follow inexorably.

Our primate cousins still share the primitive taste for

sweet foods (though they are a miniscule part of total food intake). Indeed because they enjoy certain sweet fruits, monkeys and apes in captivity have been made unhealthy by excess of these.

In the wild the odd sweet fruit might be consumed, but only as a part of a wider selection of food. Seasonal patterns would ensure that such foods were never constantly available.

Bone diseases similar to osteoporosis (common in postmenopausal Western women) have been found in monkeys fed on a diet of apples, bananas, oranges, potatoes, lettuce and carrots. When additional protein rich foods, such as eggs and liver, together with rice were added these problems ceased.

The fact that an animal 'likes' something when in an abnormal captive state does not indicate that this is all it should be fed. Nor should a child be fed on nutrient-deficient, sweetened foods, simply because it likes them.

7.
THE FIBRE-SUGAR CONNECTION

When humans live on a diet with large quantities of unrefined grains, beans, vegetables and fruit, their health is markedly better than that of those consuming few such products.

Many diseases which affect civilization, largely as a result of these dietary factors, directly involve the digestive tract. Among these are diverticular disease, constipation, appendicitis, haemorrhoids and cancer of the colon. Another problem is inadequate circulation through the pelvic area, which often leads to varicose veins and deep vein thrombosis.

These diseases are virtually unknown when unrefined foods form the major part of the diet. Refining cereals into 'white' flour, or removing the outer casing of rice to make 'white' (polished) rice, removes much of the fibre. The increased use of sugar has also reduced consumption of fibre-rich foods, such as fruits, nuts and vegetables.

Primitive cultures eat much more fibre than we do. The renowned researcher and surgeon, Denis Burkitt, spent many years in Africa, where he found that rural Africans who eat bulky fibrous foods rarely suffer from constipation, bowel cancer or appendicitis.[65] In contrast city Africans who, like American blacks and whites, eat refined foods, suffer from these diseases.

Burkitt's view is that chemicals manufactured by

bacteria in stagnant food residues, which remain for long periods in the intestines, may cause cancer in these regions. Roughage, or fibre, encourages the development of healthier intestinal bacterial flora. He also reminds us that coronary heart disease and gallstones, both linked with high blood cholesterol, are frequent in people with inadequate fibre in their diets.

FIBRE AT WORK

Foods containing fibre are more 'chewy' and so stimulate saliva production. This reduces dental problems, by neutralizing acids which form on the teeth. The extra chewing slows the rate of food intake, cuts the calories consumed, and thus reduces the overall amount of food eaten.

Refined foods require little chewing, produce little saliva and increase the acids in the mouth and the risk of decay. More food is consumed which increases overall calorie intake and the chances of obesity.

Fibre reduces cholesterol in the bloodstream and gallstone formation. It slows digestion through the small intestine and cuts the absorption of fats in this region, which is especially beneficial in overweight people. The stomach feels satisfied more easily, due to the greater bulk of high fibre foods, so there is a tendency to eat less.

In the large intestine, fibre improves bacterial cultures, inactivates some of the harmful effects of fats, improves transit time and increases the bulk of the stool, which makes its passage easier.

The risks of cancer of the colon and diverticular diseases are reduced, as are the chances of developing haemorrhoids, varicose veins and cancer of the rectum. Diabetic conditions and heart diseases are also improved or prevented by the action of fibre in the bowel.

BOWEL TRANSIT TIME

Both the bulk of stools passed and their speed of transit are dramatically improved in people on high fibre diets. Transit time is the length of time food takes to pass through the body, having been digested and with the appropriate nutrients having been extracted. In primitive tribes eating only unrefined foods, this may be as short as six hours.

Dr Andrew Stanway has described early 20th century experiments in which various foods were tested for their influence on transit time.[66] Dyes were swallowed to mark the passage of foods accurately. Barium soon became popular, since this showed up on X-ray film.

Barium scans showed that over half the subjects on a Western diet still had barium in the bowel after 48 hours; in a quarter, all the barium was still there after 72 hours; a third continued to retain some barium after five days. Rural Zulus, on the other hand, all passed all the barium within 48 hours.

More recently, opaque pellets which can be studied in detail on X-ray have been used. These, Stanway says, show that 'in most people the time that food takes to reach the colon is fairly constant, and that the majority of the 25 pellets swallowed get to the bowel all together. In the colon however the fibre content of the food really begins to take effect, and in people on high fibre foods, whether they are Africans or Westerners, the pellets pass quickly and easily through the colon and out into the stools. In those eating highly refined diets the pellets may stay in the bowel for days and become widely separated from each other. A few may even remain in the colon for a week or more.'

Ballentyne investigated the bulk of stools with comparable conclusions.[67] 'While officers in the British navy and their wives had stools which ranged in weight from 38 to 223 grams (from about two tablespoons up to a teacup in volume), British vegetarians, like the vegetarian natives of Uganda, had stools weighing from

178 to 980 grams, the average being twice that of the naval officers.'

These factors are significant in preventing many of the diseases already mentioned, most seriously cancer of the colon. This is on the increase in the West, and yet is almost unknown in underdeveloped countries. A low fibre diet is known to be a prime cause.

HOW MUCH FIBRE?

The average British and American diet contains barely 20 grams of fibre daily. NACNE urges the British public to obtain 30 grams per day, and the US Senate Select Committee recommend between 30 and 60 grams per day.

Paleolithic and modern hunter-gatherers have an intake of not less than 45 grams of fibre per day, which would effectively reduce cancer of the bowel, if followed in the West.

THE CANCER FACTOR

The bacteria in our bowels vary according to the dietary pattern of the individual. If faeces are slow in their passage through the bowel, alterations can occur in the bacterial flora of the region.

One of the major activities of the friendly bacteria which inhabit a healthy bowel is to break down the salts in the bile, so that these can be recycled for further use. A byproduct of this breakdown of bile salts is a carcinogenic substance, which is found more frequently in people with a diet low in fibre and high in fat and certain meats (notably beef).

Fibre appears to alter the function of the local bacteria and to increase the speed of transit, so that toxic material is not allowed to remain in contact with the bowel wall for long. This factor, of contact, is crucial. If transit time is measured in days, rather than hours, there is more time for harmful toxic interactions, which cause cells to become diseased and possibly cancerous.

In cases of constipation, bacteria act on fibre to produce a number of useful fatty acids. These are natural laxatives, ensuring more rapid transit time and relief of constipation.

The amount and type of fat eaten affects possible development of cancer of the colon. Too much of the wrong kind of fat combined with a low fibre diet can alter the bacterial cultures in the bowel, producing toxicity and slowing the passage of faeces. This can be disastrous.

FIBRE AND SUGAR

One of the biggest changes in the human diet over the past century has been the abandonment of high fibre foods and the adoption of ever more refined food. This includes the ubiquitous refined sugar. It is impossible to separate the implications of fibre and sugar. A high fibre diet leaves little space for refined sugar products and vice versa. It makes no difference whether sugar is white, brown or any shade between. Nutritionally there is no difference between the various types apart perhaps from the minute amounts of trace elements in dark brown sugar.

A hundred years ago sugar intake in the West was six or seven kilos per person per year, as it had been for centuries. In 1973 sugar consumption reached the highest level ever recorded of 54 kilos per man, woman and child. This has since dropped to about 38 kilos per head, which still represents some three quarters of a kilo each week. The US intake is very similar and is actually rising. As sugar intake goes up, fibre intake goes down.

NACNE strongly recommends a reduction of sugar consumption to around 20 kilos per person per year, no more than half to be derived from sweets and confectionery. This far from hopeless ideal will be more easily accomplished if high fibre is ensured in the diet. Ballentyne concludes that 'a small amount of sugar and fat in our diet, otherwise rich in proteins, vitamins and minerals, is not likely to cause trouble. In the West where

. . . refined sugar supplies 20-25% of calories, the percentage of fat in the diet may be very important. If 45% of the calories are supplied by fat and 25% by refined sugar, as is the case for the average American, then 70% of the diet is empty calories.'[68]

Empty calories are foods which supply almost nothing but calories – no minerals, no vitamins, no real nourishment. Saturated fats and sugars are both such 'non' foods. Their distortion of our diet is one of the prime causes of cancer, heart disease, arthritis and diabetes.

THE WORLD WITHIN

Our internal bacteria have an amazing turnover. A new generation comes into existence every four hours or so, the residue being excreted and forming fully one third of the stool's bulk.

When sugar is a major part of the diet, and hence fibre a small part, the bacterial and fungal colonies in the bowel develop a number of undesirable, sometimes virulent strains. These are thought to be largely responsible for the rise in cholesterol levels in the blood that have been noted on such a diet.

The NACNE report tells us that the problems of constipation and irritable bowel syndrome account for between 30% and 60% of consultations at gastroenterology clinics in Britain. The main cause, it says, is fibre deficiency.

40% of the British public believe themselves to be constipated and almost one fifth take laxatives. Cancer of the bowel is the second most common form of cancer, accounting for over 12.5% of all cancer deaths. The decline in fibre use in Britain has been rapid. Even during World War II it was between 32 and 40 grams per day, almost double current intake.

THE FIBRE-SUGAR CONNECTION

TYPES OF FIBRE

It is not only the amount, but also the type of fibre that is extremely important.

Some forms of fibre contain phytic acid, which can reduce the body's absorption of some essential minerals, especially iron and zinc, which are important in the economy of the body. Phytic acid most commonly comes from cereals, which are therefore an inferior fibre source to those found in fruits, vegetables and pulses.

These latter 'softer' types of fibre are the pectins, gums and mucilages. The cruder fibre of cereals, such as cellulose or lignin, passes through the bowel virtually unchanged and it is the action of bacteria on such fibre that often results in gaseous bloating. Bran is another such fibre and has this effect on many people, as well as its laxative function.

Ideally a high fibre diet should include a selection of vegetable foods with some crude fibre. NACNE suggests vegetable fibre should provide 12 grams per day, fruit 3 grams and the rest should be cereal fibre. Professor Stewart Trusswell has pointed out that while wheat fibre has no effect on cholesterol levels, 'viscous types (like pectin and guar) in large doses produce major reductions'.[69]

Since fresh fruits and vegetables are about 1% pectin, four portions will produce about 5 grams of pectin daily. This also reduces the intake of fats and sugar, since there is less appetite for snacks and fats.

Trusswell suggests four servings of fruit and vegetables daily. One serving should be chosen from dark green, yellow or orange foods (e.g. leafy greens, carrots, apricots, melon), and one from citrus, tropical or berry fruits, or tomatoes. Two can be selected from any other fruits or vegetables.

The remaining fibre would come from cereals and pulses. Stone Age people derived all their fibre from an enormous vegetable intake, consuming little if any cereal. The difficulties caused by excessive bran ingestion show this is not a food humans were accustomed to in prehistory. Just adding a bran supplement will not provide this basic body need.

CEREALS AND ALLERGY

Professor John Yudkin maintains that the human body is not adapted for the consumption of cereals, whether refined or unrefined.[70]

People did not consume cereal grains in any quantity until some 10,000 years ago, although some 'grass' and cereal seeds were included in their food gathering previous to this. There is evidence of wild cereals being consumed in Iraqi, Kurdistan and South Jordan in the late Stone Age, around 14,500 years ago.

The development of agriculture seems to have occurred in those regions where wild cereals were previously eaten. Tel Mureybit, in Syria, contains remains of wild cereals from 8,000 BC, about the time that cultivation of grain crops began. That is too recent for the human body to have fully adapted to cereals.

A great many people are sensitive to cereals which are a major cause of allergy. Along with the other newcomer to our diets, milk and its products, cereals should be considered as peripheral to a Stone Age eating pattern and certainly never a major part of it.

The problem seems to be that there are factors in grains, more in some than others, which create biochemical difficulties. Rice and millet are better tolerated by most people than is wheat and its products.

Clinical ecologists suggest a simple method of unearthing foods to which we may be sensitive or allergic. These are often the ones we crave for. It is as if, by having a constant intake of such foods, we suppress the acute reaction which might arise were we to avoid that food for a while and then eat it again. This phenomenon of 'masked allergy' is widespread and dairy produce and cereals figure large among the known culprits.

Fibre checklist

VERY HIGH FIBRE	PERCENTAGE FIBRE CONTENT (BY WEIGHT)	HIGH FIBRE	PERCENTAGE FIBRE CONTENT (BY WEIGHT)
Wheat bran	44.0	Hazelnuts	6.8
All bran	26.0	Barley	6.5
Apricots (dried)	24.0	Currants	6.5
Coconut (dessicated)	23.5	Spinach (boiled)	6.3
Figs (dried)	18.5	Garden peas	6.3
Prunes	16.1	Sweetcorns (kernels)	5.7
Passion fruit	15.0	Brown rice	5.5
Almond	14.3	Walnuts	5.2
Coconut (fresh)	13.5	Chick peas/	
Weetabix	12.7	Garbanzos (cooked)	5.2
Soya bean flour	12.0	Lemons	5.2
HIGH FIBRE		MEDIUM FIBRE	
Crispbread (rye)	11.7	Celeriac (boiled)	4.9
Pasta (wholewheat)	10.0	Broad beans (boiled)	4.2
Wholemeal flour	9.6	Broccoli tips (boiled)	4.1
Brazil nuts	9.0	Leeks (boiled)	3.9
Bread (wholewheat)	8.5	Spring greens (boiled)	3.8
Redcurrants	8.2	Olives	3.5
Peanuts	8.1	Cabbage (raw)	3.4
Peanut butter	7.6	Runner beans (boiled)	3.4
Wholemeal flour (85%)	7.5	Watercress	3.3
Dates	7.5	French beans	3.2
Raspberries	7.4	Carrots (raw)	2.9
Blackberries	7.3	Cabbage (boiled)	2.7
Baked beans	7.3	Carrots (boiled)	2.7
Oatmeal (raw)	7.0	Mushrooms (raw)	2.5
Sultanas	7.0	Green figs	2.5
Raisins	6.8	Apples	2.4
Chestnuts	6.8	Bananas	2.0

8.
ESSENTIAL NUTRIENTS

CALCIUM AND PHOSPHORUS

One of the most important elements in the body is calcium. Together with magnesium it is vital for cardiovascular health. Bones and teeth depend upon it for structural integrity. The nervous system needs calcium for normal transmission of impulses.

In a healthy adult, 20% of the total bone calcium is reabsorbed and replaced each year. This is called 'bone remodelling' and, for the bone structure to be maintained, the calcium which is constantly removed must be replaced in the diet. When replacement is inadequate, serious problems arise.

It is now known for certain that a high protein diet, which contains overall nutrient imbalances, can speed up the removal of calcium from bones, resulting in osteoporosis (fragile bones). Many factors contribute towards this, in particular an imbalance in the ratio of calcium to phosphorus in the diet. Phosphorus is found in very large quantities in meat and in most other proteins.

Stone Age people ate abundant meat, as do current hunter-gatherers, and yet the bone structures of both remain sound into old age. In this lies an apparent paradox – that Stone Age people did not become calcium deficient, as do so many people on a modern high protein diet. As Eaton and Konner inform us, 'Neanderthals and

Cro Magnons, who inhabited subarctic Eurasia . . . had massive bones, indicating that they obtained adequate calcium.'[71] This was despite about 35% of their diet deriving from meat, compared to under 12% of the modern diet.

FACTORS IN CALCIUM LOSS

The complex process which occurs when a high protein diet is consumed has been linked to excess of acidity caused by the protein in the body. This increases parathyroid hormone production and thus absorption of calcium from bone. Additional vitamin D can limit this progression. The body can make its own vitamin D when sufficient sunlight is available to it. Abundant exercise also appears to prevent decalcification.

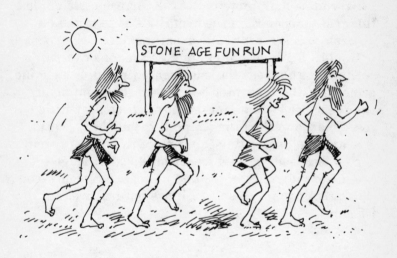

The lifestyle of our Stone Age ancestors ensured that they had abundant exercise and exposure to sunshine, and this may partly account for their not suffering decalcification. The message for us is that exercise taken in an environment where light is available is important. Direct sunlight is not necessary, as even indirect daylight has beneficial effects in the production of vitamin D.

Other possible reasons for differences in response to high protein diets relate to the levels of sugar in the blood. Increased sugar in the blood causes a decrease in the circulation of vitamin D, which combats decalcification. As the presence of high levels of sugar in the blood is directly related to the quantity of sugar eaten, this was clearly not a problem for Stone Age people.

PHOSPHORUS: THE KEY FACTOR

Demineralization of bones ceases and bone begins to remineralize when the ratio of calcium to phosphorus is 1.0 (one part of calcium for every part of phosphorus). Commonly the diet in Western society achieves a ratio of less than 0.5 (one part of calcium to two parts of phosphorus).

So while a high protein diet can increase calcium loss, this really depends on the overall balance of the diet.

A common error in many experiments which appeared to implicate a high protein diet as the major cause of calcium loss has been the use of concentrated, often liquid, proteins of the type often used in crash slimming or emergency refeeding programmes. These bear little resemblance to the forms of protein found in a natural diet and are unsafe if used for more than a very short time. Most leading researchers now acknowledge there is a major difference in the findings of experiments using such proteins and those which use natural protein foodstuffs.

ALKALINITY

Phosphorus is thought to be useful and necessary to balance the acid side effects of high protein. With phosphorus and calcium in good balance, the high vegetable content of a Stone Age diet also ensures lowered acidity contributing towards actual calcium replenishment.

Nutritional authorities such as Professor Jeffrey Bland insist that in order to achieve a reversal of bone decalcification, an alkaline-producing diet, rich in vegetable foods, is necessary.[72] This is easily achieved by those who choose vegetarianism.

If the vegetarian content approaches the levels consumed by current hunter-gatherer peoples, it is also more than adequate. In such diets, Eaton and Konner found that every 100 grams of vegetables eaten included an average of 102.5 mg of calcium, which resulted in an intake of around 1500 mg of calcium daily, just from vegetables.[73] Some game, such as venison, contains as much as 10 mg of calcium per 100 grams, which means that the total Paleolithic calcium intake was more than double that current in America and Europe, and considerably higher than the recommendations of the Senate committee.

Some of the best sources of calcium are green leafy vegetables such as dandelion greens, mustard greens, turnips and beet tops, watercress, broccoli and kale.

THE ROLE OF SODIUM

There was no known use of salt in Paleolithic times. The modern diet has, however, increased salt intake dramatically, and this has been related to conditions including high blood pressure and cancer. The link between salt intake and disease is not a direct one of cause and effect, at least in the case of high blood pressure, but depends upon imbalance between sodium, the major element of salt, and potassium, an element with which sodium has strong relationship. High intakes of sodium lead to a depletion of potassium.

Sodium is an essential element and, together with potassium, is required for normal growth and development. Sodium is involved with the body's fluid balance and so its heat control mechanism. It also helps maintain other minerals, such as calcium, in a fluid state and is important in the function of nerves and muscles.

Sodium deficiency has been connected to impaired carbohydrate metabolism and neuralgia.

BLOOD PRESSURE

Sodium influences blood pressure by reducing fluid excretion through the kidneys and by increasing the constriction of the smooth muscles which surround the tiny arteries of the body. The increased fluid retained and the more restrictive force on the blood vessels combine to cause high blood pressure. With over 95,000 kilometres of blood vessels in the body, it follows that increased pressure on a sizable part of this network will influence the overall pressure required to maintain circulation throughout.

It is also thought likely that sodium increases the activity of a hormone called angiotensin which is normally active during times of stress, when blood pressure is automatically raised to cope with increased demands for blood as the body prepares for action.

High blood pressure is the major contributory factor to the development of cardiovascular disease, the single biggest killer in the western world.

THE POTASSIUM LINK

In populations where the average blood pressure is low, sodium intake via salt is usually moderate but that of potassium is high. Potassium appears to offer a strong protective influence against the high blood pressure caused by sodium.

The ratio between sodium and potassium is now known to be more important than the actual quantities ingested – a diet high in sodium does not automatically cause high blood pressure. Evidently potassium has the effect of increasing the elimination of sodium from the body.

QUANTITIES COMPARED

Eaton and Konner found that the main vegetable foods eaten by modern hunter-gatherers contain roughly 10 mg of sodium and 550 mg of potassium in every 100 gram portion. This would amount to some 8,000 mg of potassium and 150 mg of sodium daily.

Meat would add a further 70 mg of sodium and nearly 400 mg of potassium per 100 grams, making the total Paleolithic intake approximately 700 mg of sodium with a ratio of potassium to sodium of 16.0 (16 parts of potassium for every part of sodium eaten). This appears a good ratio to follow.

Modern hunter-gatherers rarely eat more then 5 grams of salt daily. The average is around 2 grams among Eskimos and Pacific Island villagers. This translates into between 800 and 2000 mg of sodium, since salt is not all sodium.

Each gram of salt contains 400 mg of sodium. Modern man in Europe, the USA and Japan consumes vast amounts of salt, often 10 or 12 grams daily of sodium. Where these intakes are highest, the incidence of cardiovascular disease, cancer and arthritis are also highest.

CAUSE AND EFFECT

Sodium does not 'cause' these diseases directly but, as in so many disease processes, is one of many interacting factors which produce a particular disease pattern in one person and another disease in someone with different inherited and acquired characteristics.

Sodium encourages high blood pressure through alterations in the metabolism when there exists a genetically acquired susceptibility. For reasons which are not clear, black people are more prone than others.

Hypertension is often experienced in later life by children with an early exposure to high levels of sodium in the diet. This may derive from cows' milk, which has a far higher sodium level than does breast milk.

Almost all processed or preserved commercial foods have a high sodium content, unless there is a clear declaration to the contrary on the pack. It is also now known that a diet which contains appreciable amounts of sugar, or sugar-rich food, aggravates the effects of sodium. When both sugar and salt are high in the diet, blood pressure increases dramatically.

Stone Age people did not eat sugar and their sodium intake was low. We can follow their example by using a variety of condiments and herbs as salt alternatives. Pharmacies and health stores sell salt substitutes which are based on potassium chloride.

SALT IN HISTORY AND NATURE

The common root for many modern languages, Sanskrit, has no word for salt. Ballentyne suggests that at the time Indo-Europeans migrated into Europe they had not developed the custom of using salt. By Roman times, however, it was quite commonly in use. The first known salt mine is in the Austrian Tyrol and dates back to 1,000 BC.

Those primitive tribes who did use salt as a food preservative, such as the native Americans, carefully soaked the food in order to remove it before preparing food for consumption.

It has been suggested that the consumption of salt is a natural phenomenon, since animals are at times seen to lick salt. However, most animals do not adopt this strange habit, and those that do have probably acquired the taste much as man has done.

There is no physiological need for the inclusion of salt in the diet of any animal or man. When massive dietary imbalances arise, bizarre requirements for sodium may lead to salt craving. This is far from a normal, natural requirement.

COMPARATIVE SALT HABITS

Britain's National Advisory Committee on Nutritional Education (NACNE) points out that there is no hypertension in indigenous tribal societies. Typical examples are the Yanomamo Bushmen and the Samburu. These peoples' lifestyles ensure high levels of physical activity and their diets are low in animal fats and sodium. Obesity is not found amongst these peoples.

NACNE cites animal studies which prove a direct link between sodium intake and hypertension. In human studies reduced sodium or raised potassium intake were both accompanied by drops in blood pressure. Studies of over 25 different population groups have shown a direct connection between blood pressure levels and salt intake.

Finally they point out that there are no known groups of people with high average blood pressure who do not add salt to their food.

NACNE AND WHO RECOMMENDATIONS

About 20% of the population is thought to be particularly sensitive to salt.

The current intake of salt in Britain is around 12 grams per day, containing around 5 grams (5,000 mg) of sodium. In the USA the sodium intake is between 2,300 and 6,900 milligrams per day (derived from other foods as well as salt).

NACNE suggests that salt intake should be reduced to between 3 and 6 grams daily. The World Health Organisation (WHO) recommends 5 grams per day of salt (i.e. 2 grams of sodium). The US Senate committee would have its citizens reduce their intake to between 1100 and 3300 mg of sodium per day.

QUITTING THE SALT HABIT

Those who regularly sprinkle salt on their food may need to curb an habitual action as much as a desire for salt.

Cost of winter?

By blocking up most of the holes of a salt container, or by using a salt substitute, the habit is maintained but sodium consumption is greatly reduced.

Most processed food contains much hidden salt, and should be avoided whenever possible. This includes almost all canned food, much frozen food and many other items. The most enormous salt content is found in processed or preserved fish and meat products such as bacon, ham, luncheon meats, sausages, smoked or cured meats and corned beef. All pastes, relishes and sauces are high in salt, as are snack foods such as potato crisps and salted nuts. Cheese is usually a high salt food, as are soya sauces, and all foods in which baking soda has been employed. Pizza, hamburgers, hot dogs and similar 'fast foods' from modern high speed catering establishments are also very salt rich.

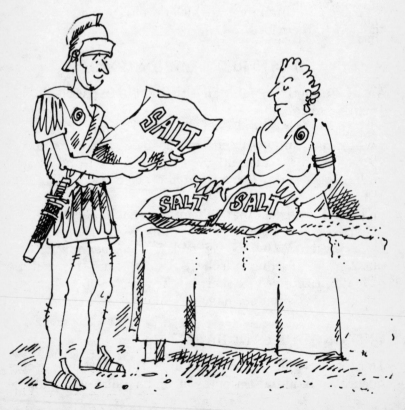

In the kitchen, the addition of salt to food when it is being cooked should be replaced by the use of culinary herbs and spices. No salt should be added at table, and above all it should be stopped in children's feeding. Many baby and infant formulas contain sodium (chemical symbol Na). Parents should look out for this and avoid such foods. New low-salt versions of many foods are appearing in response to consumer demand. It is the purchasing power of the public which can dictate a change in commercial practices, and added salt relates largely to commercial considerations. Salt has a preservative as well as a flavouring effect, but there are safer alternatives. The shelf-life of a food should not be a concern. Rather we should be concerned with our own life expectancy.

In Roman times the armies were paid in salt, the origin of the word salary. The price paid for this 'salary' in modern societies, with its consequences of disease and disability, is vast indeed.

Checklist of major nutrients in foods

FOOD		SODIUM (Na)	POTASSIUM (K)	RATIO Na/K	CALCIUM (Ca)	PHOSPHORUS (P)	RATIO Ca/P
Almonds	80 nuts	7 mg	800 mg	0.01	220 mg	490 mg	0.45
Apple	1 med	1	130	0.01	8	10	0.80
Avocado	½ med	4	604	0.01	10	42	0.24
Beans (green)	cup	6	180	0.03	60	45	1.33
Cabbage (raw)	cup	17	195	0.09	50	20	2.50
Carrots (raw)	1 lge	46	340	0.14	36	36	1.00
Cucumber	1 med	8	160	0.05	16	20	0.80
Eggs	2 hard	130	140	0.93	60	230	0.26
Halibut	100 gm	125	460	0.27	18	235	0.08
Olives	12 med	1800	42	42.86	48	12	4.00
Onion	½ cup	7	120	0.06	24	30	0.80
Peas	100 gm	230	95	2.42	26	70	0.37
Potato	1 baked	4	503	0.01	9	65	0.14
Rice (brown)	⅔ cup	265	65	4.08	12	70	0.17
Rice (white)	⅔ cup	350	25	14.00	11	28	0.39
Shrimps	100 gm	115	185	0.62	70	195	0.36
Spinach	2 cups	80	500	0.16	100	56	1.79
Tomato	1 small	3	270	0.01	15	30	0.50
Turnips	⅔ cup	36	190	0.19	35	24	1.46
Turkey	100 gm	85	400	0.21	10	280	0.04
Vegetables	⅔ cup	55	200	0.28	25	60	0.42
Walnuts	30	0	420	0.00	60	350	0.17
Pork	100 gm	1110	330	3.33	12	225	0.05

The ratio between sodium and potassium (Na/K) is arrived at by dividing the weight of sodium in a particular quantity of that food by the weight of potassium in the same quantity. Likewise the calcium/phosphorus (Ca/P) ratio is the calcium content divided by the phosphorus.

For health benefits the higher the sodium/potassium ratio the worse it is for the body (more sodium and less potassium). The lowest ratios of sodium to potassium in these examples (and therefore the best foods) were found in almonds, apples, avocados, beans, cabbage, carrots, onions, potatoes, tomatoes, spinach, turnips and walnuts (which have no sodium at all).

The higher the ratio between calcium and phosphorus, the better it is for the body (more calcium and less phosphorus). The ideal is to achieve a ratio of 1.0 (i.e the same amounts of each) in one's overall diet. Beans, cabbage, carrots, olives, spinach and turnips all provide a calcium to phosphorus ratio better than 1.0.

OTHER COMMON DEFICIENCIES

Virtually all industrialized societies show a wide range of subclinical deficiencies of essential nutrients. They appear among the young, the middle-aged and the elderly, the poor and the affluent, the pregnant and the infirm. They are found among agricultural populations in underdeveloped countries too.

As Eaton and Konner point out, the diet of Paleolithic man was adequate in providing these nutrients so commonly deficient in our societies.[74] Iron, folic acid and vitamin B12 are quoted as examples. There are differing estimates as to the true nature of deficiency in Western society. Professor Emeritus Emanuel Cheraskin claims his extensive research proves that in all sections of American society, from the affluent to those living below the poverty line, a majority are deficient in one or more major nutrient substances (vitamins, minerals, enzymes or trace elements).[75]

While other factors are, of course, involved the nutritional factors which play a part in the causation of disease are fundamental because they are by far the easiest elements to change. Altering genetic characteristics may become possible but is hardly a self-help operation. Environmental factors like pollution and stress from society's social and political upheavals are equally difficult to alter. On the other hand good food, hygiene and clean water are within our sphere of influence and play a large part in determining our state of health. Lifestyle factors such as the amount of exercise, sleep or relaxation we obtain, and whether or not we smoke or consume alcohol, all contribute towards disease and degeneration.

Other factors are involved, but poor nutritional patterns almost inevitably lead to disease regardless of these. A sound diet protects against many of the other disease-inducing factors, in relation to both physical and mental illness.

TIME FOR CHANGE?

It would probably require a cataclysmic occurrence to force people to alter their eating patterns drastically en masse. We need only consider the example of smoking and health: despite incontrovertible proof, a large body of people refuses to accept the evidence, or accepts it but continues to smoke.

Nevertheless, change has started. In just a decade there have been radical changes in the eating habits of nations such as the American and British. An accelerating trend towards vegetarianism has overtaken both nations, especially in the 18 to 30 age group. Meat consumption is dropping. Sugar consumption is down in Britain. Consumption of wholemeal bread is rising dramatically, with a corresponding drop in white flour products.

Major supermarket chains are carrying health foods and making advertising capital out of the removal of foods with additives. The number of health food shops is increasing at an astonishing rate (although some sell rather dubious products). Government and medical authorities have pronounced on the urgency of a change in Britain's diet. The World Health Organization and the US Senate Committee have made recommendations about diet which conform to views that, until only a decade or so ago, would have been held only by so-called fringe groups and cranks. The media have caught up with these trends, and feature regular comment and articles on the need for dietary change, 'alternative' healing in health care, exercise, and so on.

The impossible has begun to happen in some areas of disease as well, it seems. Through these changes there has been a notable decline in the increase of cardiovascular disease, in the USA. The USA is at least ten years ahead of Europe in this respect, and similar trends should soon be reflected in Europe's health statistics. Still, a quarter of a million people under the age of 50 in the USA will die of cardiovascular-related diseases this year. And despite the progress regarding cardiovascular disease in the USA, other major killer diseases have not yet been checked. Cancer in particular has continued to increase. It is now medically accepted that more than three quarters of all cancers have roots in nutritional factors.

There is nothing inevitable about this. Societies in which a Stone Age diet was, or is, eaten have never known these chronic diseases.

9.
THE STONE
AGE DIET

In 1977, after over fifty distinguished and successful years of treatment of disease by nutritional methods, Dr Boris Chaitow gave his views of man's diet, past and present.[76]

'Let us consider what nature and biology intended for human consumption. Before man, in his evolution, had reached a point of civilised ingenuity, when he devised the ability to create fire, his food was natural, was not refined, or purified, or whitened, or preserved, or chemicalized. But today he has literally mutilated his nutrition to the point where it is truly no wonder that he is suffering the penalties for transgressing the laws of nature. In fact it borders on a miracle that he survives at all. Surely it is a compliment to the adaptability of a living organism to be able to tolerate so much and still survive.

'When man was evolving, in distant history, his nutrition consisted of fruits, nuts, whole cereals, vegetation, roots, herbs, possibly small living creatures, etc. All nutritionally whole, all rich in the essential factors that the body requires for high efficiency, energy and freedom from disease – especially amino acids, mineral salts, trace elements, vitamins, enzymes and above all the essence and electricity of life itself. Man is the only animal in the world which tries to feed a living organism with dead food, and if you think that an

127

exaggeration, consider the nature of the Western diet in today's society. Excessive in high animal proteins, cooked, rich and fatty; a high level in starches, largely derived from refined ingredients, such as white bread, cakes, biscuits, pastries, puddings, pies, as well as white sugar, sweets, chocolates, preserves and jams, cooked, refined porridge, processed cereals, white rice or ice cream. Fluids from tea, coffee, cocoa, alcohol and synthetic and artificially sweetened bottled drinks; fried, pickled, preserved, cured, smoked, salted and tinned meats and fish; dairy products, pasteurized, homogenized and distorted by over-concentrated extractions. All of which contribute to the noxious encumbrances and the deficiencies responsible for today's tragic state of ill health. And on top of that many other items of civilized food are doctored by colouring, flavouring, preserving, sweetening, salting, chemicalizing and generally overcooking to create foodless material, that in laboratory experiments causes rats to lose their hair and teeth, to abort their young, to become irritable, pugnacious and cannibalistic, and in ludicrous seriousness causes humans to become pouchy, grouchy with falling hair, rotting teeth, poached-egg eyes, pickled livers, bleeding piles, and no idea what eating is all about.'

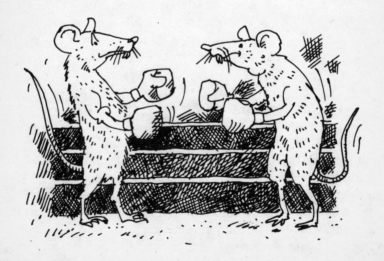

THE IMPORTANCE OF DIET

The food we eat is a major, and some would say *the* major, factor in determining our level of health and well-being. It is also a major factor influencing the way we die, and the degree of discomfort associated with this inevitable process.

Inborn genetic factors, interacting with our nutritional status, are the two basic elements which determine health. We can at present do little regarding genetic characteristics, but diet offers a chance for positive action and acceptance of responsibility for our state of health. This is not to deny the importance of other mental, emotional and physical factors in the causation of disease, nor to negate the value of treatment for ill health. But our concern, and the keystone of healthcare, is the prevention of ill health. Diet is the means.

Each individual must choose his or her own mode of eating. From a health viewpoint, the vegetarian way is potentially superior to current dietary patterns. It also carries with it certain ethical, compassionate and spiritual overtones which make it appealing to many. However, for those who wish to avoid the excesses of modern food production and seek a healthier lifestyle,

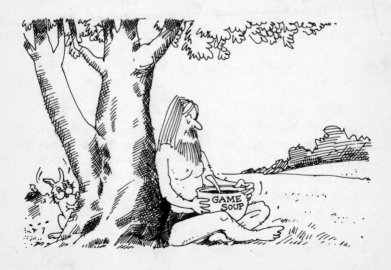

but who are reluctant to avoid the eating of meat, the Paleolithic pattern is an alternative.

We will now summarise the findings made in this exploration of the Stone Age diet, and make suggestions as to the eating patterns which they indicate for modern society. We will also list some of the foods and 'non' foods which are so much a part of modern life and yet foreign to us in so far as they are recent additions to our diets.

Milk and diary produce are of particular concern since they play an enormous part in the modern diet. That no allergic reaction has been experienced in itself is not sufficient reason for assuming that dairy products should therefore be incorporated, ad lib, into the diet. Fat, for example, is very much a part of the problem with milk products. In terms of food value, low-fat yoghurts represent a reasonable compromise. In addition low-fat cheese, such as cottage cheese or Dutch Edam, or cheese made from goats' or sheep's milk, such as the Greek Feta, are preferable to high-fat cheeses.

There are also a number of soured or cultured milk products which have been found useful in certain health conditions, including acidophilus milk and kefir. Products with a culture incorporated into their basic dairy food content, such as natural yoghurt and sour milk, are helpful in restoring the health of bowel flora, especially if antibiotics have been used at any time. None of these are part of the true Stone Age diet, but represent a degree of modification which is acceptable so long as there is no known sensitivity or allergy to dairy foods.

Cereals present a similar problem in that they are ubiquitous and very hard to avoid. However we were not designed to consume them in any quantity, and the best advice is that cereals and flour products be avoided wherever possible, ideally abandoned, and certainly limited to a very minor part of the diet.

We do not require bread for health. Man survived extremely well without it, or any other cereal products, for hundreds of thousands of years. Allergies to cereals are widespread, a fact which should be borne in mind if there is any craving for such a food, as this is often an indication of such a sensitivity.

Meat should play a major part in Stone Age eating, unless a vegetarian food pattern is chosen. The meat which is eaten should not include any from farm-raised cows, pigs, sheep or other domesticated animals.

Game is acceptable for such a diet. In its broad sense, game means any animal, bird or fish which has grown as in the wild.

Chicken and other poultry should be avoided, unless truly free range, that is from birds which have lived freely out of doors, finding their own food. Birds which have been fed on commercial preparations of poultry food are not acceptable in a Stone Age diet.

Fish forms part of Stone Age dietary content if it is from free-living sea or river fish. Fish from polluted areas should be avoided.

Eggs played a marginal part in the diet of Stone Age people. They did not keep birds, but consumed eggs when and if they came across them. This is also true of the great apes. Therefore the use of eggs in moderation is acceptable as part of a Stone Age eating pattern, provided there is no allergy to them (eggs are a common source of allergy). One egg a day, again from truly free range birds, would seem reasonable.

Sugar is not a part of Stone Age eating, and there are no exceptions to this, apart from a honey 'treat' from time to time.

Salt is not necessary. In cooking it can be replaced, when a salty taste is desired, by the use of potassium chloride. Other condiments, herbs and spices are acceptable in moderation. Sodium is sufficiently present in food naturally to ensure that deficiency will not occur.

Tea and coffee are not a part of Stone Age eating patterns and are not recommended. Herbal teas often contain the same elements known to be undesirable in tea and coffee. There are a few 'safe' herbal teas, which include rooibos (red bush), camomile and linden flower. The decaffeination of coffee or tea does not remove other undesirable elements. Indeed some methods of decaffeination actually increase the toxicity of the final product.

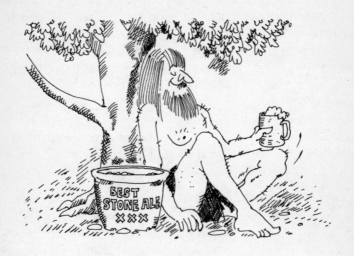

Alcohol is destructive of life and health. Its use is not recommended but this will not stop some people. In such cases, alcohol intake should be limited to wine or beer and should not exceed one or one and a half glasses of white wine daily, or a half pint of real ale. Spirits should never be consumed.

Processed foods of all sorts are not Stone Age foods. In this category are included all canned foods and anything which contains additives, be they preservatives, colouring, stabilizers or any other of the multitude of substances used to 'improve' products. They do not improve the quality of food in nutritional terms. Margarine and other processed oils and fats should be avoided.

Foods which are not included in the Stone Age diet

- Milk from any animal except human*
- Any of the products of milk*
- All cereals and their products†
- Sugar in any form
- Meat from domesticated animals (pigs, cows, sheep, etc.)
- Chicken unless free range
- Eggs unless free range
- Alcohol ‡
- Coffee, tea and related beverages
- All manufactured foods (canned, bottled, etc.)
- All processed meat or fish (smoked, pickled, salted, etc.)
- Chocolate and cocoa products

*Modification of the Stone Age diet includes natural (live) low-fat yoghurt and cultured milk products in moderation.
†The cereals which are best tolerated are rice and millet.
‡If unavoidable a little dry white wine or real ale is acceptable.

Foods which make up the Stone Age diet

- All fruit§
- All game and fish‖
- Free range eggs
- All vegetables
- Some herb teas
- All fresh nuts

§Citrus fruits upset some people, and should be used with caution by those with sensitivities and allergies.
‖Not when a vegetarian diet has been selected.

Water The water which emerges from taps, especially in industrialized areas and cities, is frequently recycled and commonly contains huge amounts of undesirable material, such as heavy metals, petro-carbon traces and various chemicals. The chemicals used in 'cleaning' this, such as chlorine, are highly undesirable. It is therefore suggested that water from a safe source, such as spring water, be used for drinking purposes. For those who are particularly sensitive, it should also be used for cooking.

ORGANIC PRODUCE

The trend towards organic production of crops is rising. Major supermarket chains are now marketing organically grown vegetables and fruits, and many small greengrocers can supply these foods, which are free of chemicals. Every effort should be made to obtain such supplies in place of products which have had a variety of chemicals added to the soils in which they grow or sprayed onto them.

While the cosmetic appearance of organic foods is not always the same as that of commercial produce – there may not be a uniformity of size in tomatoes or a waxy sheen on apples – the nutritive value is superior.

BALANCE, QUANTITIES AND RATIOS IN NUTRIENTS

Protein This should form anything from 12 to 20% of the diet. In Stone Age times this came almost entirely from meat and comprised 34% of the total energy intake. Current levels in the USA and Europe are around 12%. This should be maintained or increased, either through greater use of game and fish, or by an increase in vegetarian protein.

Additional vitamin B6 is required by individuals who eat large amounts of meat. The dietary patterns described below will provide this. However a supplement of this vitamin is suggested at a dosage of 50 mg daily if the protein intake is mainly meat-based (game).

The total intake of meat by Stone Age people was enormous – between 700 and 800 grams per person per day. Today, however, very few individuals approach the energy output of Stone Age people and a smaller intake of between 100 and 250 grams per day of food from animal source (fish, game, egg, etc.) is recommended.

Carbohydrate   Stone Age people obtained about 45% of their energy from complex carbohydrates and almost none from simple carbohydrates such as sugar. Modern man achieves a similar overall intake, but most of this is in the form of sugars.

Following a Stone Age pattern of eating will increase the intake of complex carbohydrates (unrefined, as from beans, vegetables or seeds) to a level which may approach that suggested by the McGovern Senate Select Committee of 58% of total energy intake.

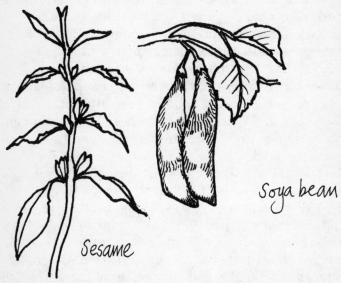

Soya bean

Sesame

If total compliance with a no-sugar injunction cannot be adhered to, sugar should only be taken rarely, as regular use will sabotage the entire health promotion plan. No single factor is more destructive of physiological function than simple sugar. It is not part of Stone Age eating and should be scrupulously avoided, especially by children.

Fats   By changing to a diet including game and fish, and by avoiding most dairy produce, domesticated animal meats and chicken skin, overall fat intake should drop dramatically from the current 41% of total energy intake (excluding alcohol) towards the ideal of under 30%. The fat content of Stone Age people represented only around 21% of their total energy intake. Current health guidelines suggest that fat should account for between 30 and 35% of total energy intake.

The ratio between polyunsaturated and saturated fats for Stone Age people was 1.41 (the amount of polyunsaturated fat in their diet divided by the amount of saturated fat). This means there was about one and a half times as much polyunsaturated fat as saturated in their diet. This is an objective to aim for. The current US ratio in these fats is 0.44, indicating that nearly twice as much saturated as polyunsaturated fat is eaten.

NACNE stress that any improvement in this ratio should not be achieved by increasing the intake of polyunsaturated oils, but rather by a reduction in saturated ones. There are risks associated with high levels of polyunsaturates too. The overall level of fats must decline, and this should be achieved by a reduction in saturated fats and a marginal increase in monounsaturated oils, such as olive oil. NACNE and WHO recommend that no more than 10% of energy intake should come from saturated fats and the McGovern Committee recommend a ratio of polyunsaturated to saturated oils of 1.00 (that is, equal quantities). As dairy fat provides roughly one third, and meat fat at least a quarter, of all saturated fat in our modern diet, a change to game and fish and the abandonment of dairy produce will achieve these goals easily and safely.

Cholesterol   There are no specific recommendations about cholesterol. The increase in fibre intake, the balance of other nutrients and the absence of sugar will ensure that naturally occurring cholesterol levels (i.e. the major part of blood cholesterol, which does not derive from food sources) will be moderate.

Cholesterol is essential for health and the dietary intake has but a marginal effect on this. Stone Age intake was similar to today's. This is roughly double the recommendation of the McGovern Committee, while NACNE makes no specific recommendations. Improvements in overall dietary balance will take care of any cholesterol problems.

Fibre Stone Age diets provide upwards of 45 grams of fibre daily. Modern diets in Europe and the USA provide around 20 grams. Various authorities recommend that this be raised to between 30 and 60 grams daily.

An increase in complex carbohydrates, which the Stone Age diet achieves automatically, will result in an increase in fibre of all sorts. This is important, as cereal fibres have limited benefit, and those gums and mucilages derived from fruits, pulses and vegetables are the most beneficial fibres for man.

Sodium No salt was added to food in the Stone Age. None is suggested for modern man. The overall sodium intake required for health, in balance with potassium, can be achieved from natural sources. Both elements are found in vegetables in desirable levels. Current intake of salt in the Western world should be reduced to between three and five grams per day maximum. Herbs, spices or a little potassium chloride, for flavouring, will compensate for the loss of salt.

Calcium The ratio of calcium to phosphorus should be about 1.0 (as much calcium as phosphorus). Current Western diets provide only about half as much calcium as they do phosphorus, in contrast to the Stone Age diet which achieved a very good ratio, with even more calcium than phosphorus in the diet. A higher ratio will automatically result if the vegetable intake, which alkalizes the bloodstream, is high enough. Bone demineralization will then cease to be a potential hazard.

Total calcium intake in Stone Age times was around 1600 milligrams per day. Ours is under 750 milligrams. Recommendations are that this should be increased to 1200 milligrams. This level will easily be achieved by following the Stone Age diet, without the need for dairy produce.

Vitamin C   Stone Age people derived some 400 milligrams of ascorbic acid from their food daily. Current levels in the USA are around 85 milligrams, and recommendations suggest a mere 45 milligrams. These recommendations take no account of the evidence presented in Chapter 5, which indicates that the Stone Age intake was approximately the right level for man.

A Stone Age eating pattern will ensure adequate vitamin C. If this cannot be followed, then supplementation at a rate of 200 to 300 mg daily is suggested.

Vitamin D and exercise   A prescription for healthy calcium levels must include adequate exercise and exposure to daylight. These were a natural and inevitable part of daily life in the Stone Age. This is not the case for most of us today, and aerobic principles should be adopted, which call for a period of brisk exercise (walking will do) at least every other day.

Other nutrients   The meat of game contains desirable substances such as eicosapentenoic acid (EPA), which is also found in edible seeds like linseed. Effectively, all nutrients (and even some which remain to be identified) will be adequately provided in a Stone Age pattern of eating. A balanced vegetarian diet will make the same provisions. All other vitamins and minerals will be similarly available, and supplementation is not suggested, unless a specific nutrient deficit is indicated.

DRINKS

A very few herb teas are known to be almost totally safe. These include the South African rooibos (red bush) tea, camomile and linden flower. Natural spring water is the best drink.

Fruit juices tend to have an imbalancing effect on blood sugar, because of the concentrated manner in which the fruit sugars reach the digestive system. When a fruit is eaten whole, the juice is absorbed reasonably slowly into the system. But in the absence of fibrous material and pulp, the sugar in the juice is rapidly absorbed, increasing the blood sugar level and causing rapid deployment of insulin to balance the excess sugar. This cycle of events can be damaging to the organism, so juices should be taken infrequently and sipped rather than gulped.

Alcohol consumption should be minimal: one and a half glasses of dry white wine daily or a half pint glass of real beer is a suggested limit.

VEGETARIAN CONSIDERATIONS

Those who choose the vegetarian option must pay special attention to adequate protein intake. A combination of seeds and pulses, or occasionally grains and pulses, at the same meal will provide a complement of amino acids, which the body can turn into first class protein. This replaces the first class protein in meat, which has been synthesized from vegetables by the animal.

While quantities are impossible to recommend, at least one main meal a day should include a large portion of a seed and pulse, or grain and pulse, combination. If the vegetarian also includes eggs and a certain amount of acceptable low-fat dairy produce in the diet, this critical factor of amino acid combinations becomes less vital.

Still, the single most undesirable aspect of many vegetarian diets is their failure to achieve adequate protein intake, and consequent dependence on carbohydrates. The eating of a seed, fruit and nut-based breakfast, as described in the suggested vegetarian menu below, will considerably boost protein intake.

SEASONAL INFLUENCES

It has long been a principle of macrobiotic feeding that only fruits and vegetables in season, and only those indigenous to the area, should be eaten. This has a philosophical niceness and appeals to a sense of order in the universe and nature. It also assumes that man is in fact living where nature intended him to live.

Certainly there is a degree of manipulation of fruits and vegetables in order to get them in a fit state to markets across the world. Domestic produce is more likely to have been picked at a stage of ripeness which is consonant with nutritional perfection. Local seasonal fruits and vegetables are therefore recommended. A certain degree of licence, however, is suggested with tropical fruits, which are as close as most of us will ever get to the tropical jungles of our origins.

COOKED OR RAW

Whether a vegetarian or a meat-based diet is followed, a balance of two thirds raw and one third cooked is suggested. This balance has been found ideal by many nutritionists for health maintenance and enhancement.

An absolute minimum of half cooked and half raw should be adhered to, and a higher intake of raw food attempted if possible.

SUGGESTED MENU: VEGETARIAN OPTION

Breakfast   Choose from
   natural low fat yoghurt
   seed and nut mixture (see recipe in following chapter)
   fresh fruit
   egg
   drink of herb tea

Midmorning/Midafternoon snack   Seeds, nuts and/or fruit.

Main meals   One of the main meals for the vegetarian should be raw and the other cooked. The ideal of two thirds raw will be achieved by this pattern, with one cooked and one raw main meal, and the breakfast described above.

The raw meal should be a large mixed salad, with as many varieties of available cultivated and free-growing ingredients as possible. There should be daily servings of wide-leafed, dark green vegetables and yellow or orange coloured vegetables (pumpkin, squash, carrot), plus at least two portions from other sources (tomato, potato, etc.). This should achieve a variety of tastes and textures as well as colours, so that the eye and palate do not become bored. With the salad have an assortment of nuts and seeds and/or a baked potato, plus cottage cheese, avocado or feta cheese. Dress the salad with lemon juice and olive oil or yoghurt. Dessert can be fresh fruit or nuts.

The cooked main meal should combine pulses (chickpeas, butter beans, haricot beans, mung beans, lentils, etc.) and seeds (sunflower, pumpkin, sesame, etc.). This combination may take the form of a soup, a 'nutroast', a vegetable stew, or any other form your ingenuity can devise. If grains are included (a personal decision) then rice, wheat or millet can be combined with pulses to create the complete amino acid complement required for the synthesizing by the body of a first-class protein. Cooking methods are important, and steaming or stir frying are best. Roasting and deep frying tend to alter the fat content and are inferior forms of cooking. Baking and cooking in a casserole are also acceptable methods, but the boiling of vegetables tends to diminish their nutrient value, unless cooking is only for a short time. The water used in boiling vegetables can be beneficially consumed in soup or simply drunk, when mineral content will be very high.

SUGGESTED MENU: GAME OPTION

Breakfast Choose from
  natural yoghurt
  fresh fruit
  egg
  seed and nut mixture (see recipe in the following
  chapter)
  fish or game

Midmorning/Midafternoon snack Seeds, nuts and/or fruit.

Main meals These can be based on fish, meat or fowl
(game), or a vegetarian protein dish. Some of the
vegetables should be raw, to achieve a balance between
cooked and raw food. It is suggested that, as a matter
of habit, a side salad be included whenever meat or fish
is eaten, and that this form the bulk of the vegetable
component. Some cooked vegetables are of course both
desirable and permissible.

Non-vegetarians should attempt to cultivate a taste for
some of the vegetarian possibilities and should periodically
include pulses, a rich source of fibre, in their diet.

As with the vegetarian diet, the vegetables and fruits
should be chosen each day from the different groups (dark
green, orange or yellow, etc.) and a wide variety of free-
growing vegetables should be consumed. These may
include mustard greens, dandelion leaves or comfrey.
Dessert should be fruit.

Detoxification is often useful when large quantities of
animal protein are consumed, especially if inadequate
raw food is eaten. On one day each week the meat eater
should eat only vegetarian foods, concentrating
particularly on raw foods. On this day fruits and salads
in the main will be consumed.

The use of garlic and onions further aids detoxification,
as these are rich in useful substances such as sulphur
and selenium. These can be eaten cooked or raw, and are
also a major help in the switch from salt to the seasoning
of food with herbs and spices.

10.
STONE AGE RECIPES

Strictly speaking, to cook in Stone Age ways would involve little more than a fire and the food. This is most closely mirrored in barbecue cooking, for which some methods are given below.

The recipes are in the main adapted from traditional Greek methods of cooking with which I am familiar. Game is still much eaten in Greece, when available, and the acceptability of free range chicken in a Stone Age diet has allowed for a number of other recipes.

Much use is made in some recipes of olive oil, which requires a degree of explanation. It is now well established that the monounsaturated oils, such as olive oil, have a better effect on cholesterol levels than the polyunsaturated oils, such as sunflower and corn oil. As long as the oil used is a virgin oil, or is cold-pressed or first-pressed, it will be a highly desirable addition to the nutrition of the body.

In cooking, oils should never reach the point of actually smoking, for this alters their chemistry. Otherwise, there is no apology required for the use of olive oil. The health of the inhabitants of Southern Europe speaks volumes for its benefits, as for those of garlic.

A number of recipes have been adapted from other sources, and I would like to pay tribute to the work of John Edwards in helping me to appreciate the amazing variations in the use of culinary herbs in ancient times.[77]

The use of some organ meats is unappealing to many. There is little logic in this since the food value of spleen or liver, for example, is far greater than that of muscle meat. I have included some recipes for these organs, as well as some traditional Greek methods for the preparation of other parts, such as the intestines and stomach. The ambitious or brave may attempt these on their unsuspecting families. The tastes may be so delicious that they outweigh any apparent squeamishness.

I have concentrated on foods and recipes that are not dealt with commonly in other books. Fish and vegetarian meals are well-covered elsewhere as are cookery books which emphasize low-fat and low-salt cooking.

ALKMINI CHAITOW
Corfu 1986

SEED AND NUT BREAKFAST

Recommended seeds include sunflower, pumpkin, linseed (flax), sesame and pine kernels. Most of these are available from healthfood or wholefood stores. Ensure that the seeds are meant for human consumption and not intended as bird seed mixture. All seeds and nuts should be fresh.

Choose three or more of the following: 1 dessertspoon sunflower seeds; 1 dessertspoon pumpkin seeds; ½ – 1 dessertspoon pine kernels; ½ – 1 dessertspoon linseed; ½ dessertspoon sesame seeds

Chopped sun-dried fruit; 30 gms of milled or grated fresh nuts (almonds, walnuts, pecans, hazelnuts, etc.); a grated apple; tropical fruit such as passion fruit, kiwi fruit or papaya

Soak the seeds in a little water overnight, then in the morning add the dried fruit and/or nuts, grated apple, and fresh tropical fruit.

If yoghurt is being included as part of a modified Stone Age diet, add this to the mixture as a dressing. Those who enjoy their food chewy and dry can omit the overnight soaking and use yoghurt to moisten the mixture.

If grains are being eaten as part of the diet, then the ingredients for overnight soaking could include flaked or whole millet or oat flakes, and the final preparation could incorporate wheatgerm.

This is a highly nutritious meal and should be well chewed. Quantities given are approximate as appetites differ, and the ingredients can be varied. Dried fruit can include apricot, peach, sultanas or dates, but ensure such fruits are really sun-dried, and not chemically dehydrated. Experiment with the ingredients and quantities, and also with the overnight soaking – this is often a matter of personal choice.

SMALL BIRDS

The following recipes are suitable for any small to medium sized birds available, such as quail, pigeon, partridge or guinea fowl. The quantities given, which provide for two generous portions, are based on pigeon, and should be amended for different-sized birds. Note that the livers and lungs of birds can also be eaten.

PIGEON IN RED SAUCE

2 birds; 1 medium onion (thinly chopped or grated); ¾ tablespoon tomato purée; ¾ teacup virgin olive oil; a little pepper; salt substitute (potassium chloride or a teaspoon of honey)

Clean and wash the birds. Place the oil in a large casserole or saucepan, then add the birds, onion, pepper and potassium chloride (if used as a salt substitute). Cook on a gentle heat, stirring constantly, until the birds are slightly browned. Add half a glass of warm water, cover and simmer for 15 minutes.

Dissolve the tomato purée (and honey, if this has been selected as a salt substitute), in two tablespoons of hot water, and add to the contents of the saucepan. If there is not sufficient liquid to cover the birds, add more water. Cover and simmer on a medium heat, stirring periodically, until most of the liquid has evaporated, leaving the birds in a small quantity of sauce.

Serve with cooked vegetables of your choice.

PIGEONS STUFFED WITH OLIVES IN WINE SAUCE

2 birds; 12 stoned black olives; 3 tablespoons virgin olive oil; 1 teaspoon dried oregano; ½ wineglass white wine; black pepper (optional); salt substitute (optional)

Mix together the oregano, olives, salt substitute and pepper to taste and place this mixture in the body cavity of each bird.

Place the oil in a large casserole or saucepan. Add the birds and cook on a low heat for a few minutes, until the skin is slightly browned. Add the wine and cook for a further five minutes. Add sufficient hot water to just cover birds and simmer until the liquid has evaporated. This will leave the birds, which should now be dark brown, in a sauce.

Serve with mixed salad and baked or mashed potato.

PIGEON SOUVLAKI

2 birds, halved; 1 green pepper sliced into 2 cm squares; 1 red pepper sliced into squares; 1 large onion, sliced; 3 small firm tomatoes, sliced; 2 teaspoons dried oregano; salt substitute; freshly ground pepper; 2 or 3 tablespoons olive oil

Place all the ingredients into a large bowl and gently but thoroughly mix this, so that the vegetables and the birds are well covered. Onto metal skewers place alternately portions of the various vegetables and the halved birds. Cook these on a hot barbecue or grill until the birds are golden brown, turning frequently. Baste the skewers from time to time with the remaining oil/oregano mixture to prevent birds from drying.

Souvlaki can also be cooked in an oven. Arrange the skewers in a shallow roasting tin. Brush lightly with the olive oil/ oregano mixture. Then add a wineglassful of water. Cook for approximately 40 minutes on a medium heat (Gas Mark 4, 180°C) or until tender, turning periodically during cooking.

PIGEON WITH GARLIC

2 birds; 12 cloves of garlic; ⅔ teaspoon oregano; salt substitute; a little pepper; olive oil

Mix oregano, pepper and salt substitute together. Place some of this mixture in the body cavity of each bird, together with the whole cloves of garlic. Using a pastry brush, coat the birds with oil, then cover with foil and place them in an oven preheated to Gas Mark 4, 180°C. Cook for approximately 40 minutes or until tender.

STIFADO

2 birds halved; 16 shallots; 1 medium-sized onion, chopped; 2–3 tablespoons olive oil; 4 bay leaves; 1 wineglass white wine; 1 tablespoon tomato purée; 2 tablespoons chopped parsley; salt substitute; freshly ground black pepper; pinch of paprika; 6 whole cloves of garlic

Place the oil in a large casserole or saucepan. Then add the birds, chopped onion, parsley, black pepper, paprika and salt substitute. Cook over a medium heat, stirring continuously until the onion is slightly browned. Add the wine, stir, and allow to cook for a further 2 to 3 minutes. Then add the bay leaves, shallots, tomato purée and enough water to cover the birds.

Cover the container and simmer gently until the birds are tender and most of the liquid has evaporated.

Serve with cooked vegetables and baked potatoes.

BARBECUED PIGEON

2 birds; 2 tablespoons lemon juice; oregano; 2 tablespoons olive oil

Mix the oil and lemon juice in a bowl. Place the washed, cleaned and dried birds into this and coat them completely in the mixture. Remove and place on a spit over a hot barbecue or under a grill. Turn frequently and baste with the remaining oil/juice mixture. Continue until the birds are golden brown.

BASIC ROASTING FOR SMALL OR MEDIUM-SIZED GAME BIRDS (QUAIL, PHEASANT, WILD DUCK, ETC.)

1 kilo bird; 1 teaspoon salt substitute; 1/4 tablespoon fennel seed; 3 turnips; 1 tablespoon olive oil; 1 tablespoon chopped chives; 1 tablespoon coriander

Simmer the bird(s) in water seasoned with salt substitute and fennel seed for half an hour. Clean the turnips and boil in a separate pan until tender. Drain off and reserve the cooking water.

Place the bird(s) in a roasting pan, with the olive oil, turnip stock, chives and coriander. Roast in a moderate oven (Gas Mark 4, 180°C) until brown and tender. Baste frequently.

SAUCES

A variety of sauces can be made to complement roast bird. These are not, of course, intended for use with recipes which produce their own sauce.

ROSEMARY SAUCE

1/2 teaspoon black pepper; 1/2 teaspoon celery seed; a few leaves of mint; 1 teaspoon rosemary; 1/2 wineglass white wine; 1 tablespoon olive oil; 1 wineglass water or vegetable stock

With a pestle and mortar grind together the pepper, celery seed, mint and rosemary. When the ingredients are well mixed, transfer them to a saucepan together with the wine, oil, and water or vegetable stock.

Simmer until reduced to a thick consistency. The birds can be braised in this during the final stages of cooking or the sauce may be added to the roasted bird.

NUT AND SAFFRON SAUCE

½ teaspoon ground black pepper; ½–1 teaspoon parsley; 1 teaspoon celery seed; ½ teaspoon chopped mint; a touch of saffron; 1 wineglass dry white wine; 2 tablespoons whole hazelnuts or almonds; 1 tablespoon honey; 1 teaspoon wine vinegar; 1 tablespoon olive oil

Lightly roast the nuts in the oven. With a pestle and mortar grind the dry ingredients (nuts, herbs, seeds and seasoning) and then add wine. Mix thoroughly and add the vinegar and honey.

Place the olive oil in a saucepan and add the mixed ingredients and one cup of water. Bring to the boil and simmer for about 20 to 25 minutes on a low heat to reduce to a thick consistency.

The sauce should be added to birds when they are nearing the completion of roasting by marking the skin with a knife and pouring the sauce over the birds, which are then cooked for a few minutes more.

'HIGH' GAME BIRDS

When birds are no longer fresh, having been hung, they can be cooked by simmering in water seasoned with half a teaspoon of fennel seed for half an hour before being placed in a roasting dish and cooked. Baste with a mixture of blended seasonings such as the following:

1 teaspoon each ground pepper, mint and thyme; ½ teaspoon celery seeds; 1½ tablespoons chopped almonds or hazelnuts; 1½ tablespoons chopped dates; 1 tablespoon each honey and wine vinegar; 1 dessertspoon olive oil; 2 wineglasses vegetable or chicken stock

Bring the mixture to the boil before pouring over the bird in the roasting tin. Baste frequently.

If game is not available, there are many suitable recipes which use free range chicken. The same recipes may also be used for medium-sized game birds.

FREE RANGE CHICKEN AVGOLEMONO

This recipe makes a tasty soup for four

1 kilo free range chicken; 5 stalks celery, including leaves; 5–6 cups rice (unpolished); 1 wineglass lemon juice; 2 eggs; salt substitute; pinch of pepper

Place the washed chicken into a saucepan. Add salt substitute and pepper, the celery (whole) and cover with water. Cook on a gentle heat for 45 minutes. If more water is required during cooking, this should be added hot so that the cooking is not interrupted.

When the chicken is tender, remove it from the pan and put it on a plate. Remove and discard the celery. Bring the cooking water back to the boil and add the rice. Boil over a medium heat, stirring occasionally, until the rice is cooked.

Meanwhile, separate the whites of the eggs from the yolks. Beat the egg whites until frothy. Then quickly but gently blend the yolks into the whites. Leave this egg mixture on one side.

When the rice is cooked, remove the saucepan from the heat. Take a cupful of the cooking liquid from the pan and add it to the lemon juice. Mix well.

Stirring constantly, alternately add to the contents of the saucepan small amounts of the egg mixture and the lemon and water mixture. Continue until all the ingredients are well mixed. Allow to stand for 5 minutes.

The rice soup can be served as a starter followed by the chicken (deboned and with appropriate vegetables or salad); alternatively the chicken meat may be removed from the bone, chopped, and added to the soup which is then served as a main course.

CHICKEN AND GINGER CASSEROLE

1½ kilo chicken or other game bird; 1 teaspoon ground black pepper; ½ teaspoon celery seeds; ¼ teaspoon caraway seeds; 1 teaspoon ginger; ½ wineglass vegetable or chicken stock; ¼ wineglass white wine; ½ wineglass hot water

Grind the dry ingredients with a pestle and mortar, and add the liquids. Place the bird in a casserole or clay cooking pot, and pour the mixture over it. Cover the container and cook until tender in an oven preheated to Gas Mark 4, 180°C for approximately 1½ hours.

CHICKEN WITH GARLIC

1 chicken weighing approximately 1 kilo; ½ kilo potatoes; 5 cloves garlic, chopped; 1 teaspoon oregano; juice of one lemon; ¾ teacup of olive oil

Wash the potatoes thoroughly, but do not peel. Cut them into quarters and place together with the well-cleaned chicken into a shallow casserole or roasting tin. Over this spread the chopped garlic and oregano. Pour on olive oil, lemon juice and a cup of water.

Cover with foil and cook in an oven preheated to Gas Mark 4, 180°C for 1–1¼ hours. Remove the foil and cook until golden brown.

KLEFTIKO

The following recipe is especially suitable for the meat of deer, kid or wild pig (boar) and will feed up to ten people.

2 kilos meat; 1 tablespoon oregano; 1 tablespoon thyme; 1 wineglass lemon juice; salt substitute; black pepper (optional); 2 tablespoons olive oil

Mix together the olive oil, lemon juice, oregano, thyme, salt substitute and pepper. Keeping the meat in one piece, make deep cuts into it. Then rub the herb mixture over the surface of the meat.

Double wrap the meat in foil, place it in a shallow casserole or roasting tin and cook in an oven preheated to Gas Mark 4, 180°C. After 1½ hours check the meat, and if dry baste with more of the herb mixture. Rewrap and cook until pricking the meat produces no blood.

MARINATED KID

Serves four to five

1 kilo kid; 2 teaspoons ground pepper; 1½ teaspoons rosemary; 1 teaspoon thyme; 2 finely chopped onions; 2 wineglasses vegetable stock

Combine together the herbs, seasoning, onion and vegetable stock to make the marinade. Pour the marinade over the meat to cover. Leave overnight.

To cook, remove the meat from the marinade, place in a shallow casserole or roasting tin with a little olive oil, and roast in an oven preheated to Gas Mark 4, 180°C until tender.

SPICED KID

Serves four or five

1 kilo kid; 1 chopped onion; ¼ teaspoon celery seed; ½ teaspoon ground coriander; ¼ teaspoon ground cumin

Mix together the coriander, celery seed and cumin. Rub this mixture well into the portion of kid, which may first be lightly scored to aid absorption. Roast, without covering, in an oven preheated to Gas Mark 4, 180°C for approximately 2 hours, until tender.

STIFADO: FOR VENISON, RABBIT OR HARE

Serves four to five

1 kilo meat; ½ kilo shallots; 1½ dessertspoons tomato purée, diluted in 2 tablespoons warm water; 10 cloves garlic (whole); 1½ wineglasses white wine; 3 tablespoons olive oil; 1 teaspoon rosemary; 4 bayleaves; salt substitute

Place the meat into a saucepan or, ideally, an earthenware pot, together with the garlic, shallots (all whole) and olive oil. Cook on a medium heat, stirring frequently. When the meat is slightly browned (after 10–15 minutes), add the wine and cook for a further 5 minutes before adding the rest of the ingredients. Cover with hot water and simmer until the meat is cooked and most of the liquid has evaporated.

HARE OR RABBIT WITH LEMON JUICE

Serves four

4 medium-sized joints of hare, cut into quarters; juice of 2 lemons; 3 tablespoons olive oil; pepper and salt substitute (optional)

Place the meat in a casserole or earthenware container, cover with water and the juice of one lemon, and stand overnight.
   Place the marinated meat in a saucepan with the oil and cook over a medium heat, turning constantly until lightly browned. Add the remaining lemon juice, a little at a time, then cover the meat with boiling water. Cover the pan and allow to simmer gently until tender. Stir occasionally and add more hot water if necessary. When tender there should be a little sauce left in the container to serve with the meat.

ORGAN MEATS

Some organ meats may be unfamiliar to the reader. Spleen, for example, is highly nutritious and is sometimes available from local butchers (calf or sheep spleen). If game spleen is available this is to be preferred.

GRILLED SPICED LIVER

Bird liver should be used whole; liver from larger animals should be sliced in 1 cm thicknesses.

The meat should be well washed and drained, then placed in a bowl containing a little olive oil. Soak for 1 hour and then grill under a gentle heat (excessive heat makes the liver harden). When cooked season with lemon juice, fresh thyme or oregano and a touch of olive oil.

SPLEEN

The spleen of any animal may be used. Two lamb spleens or one calf spleen would be sufficient for a single portion. A deer's spleen might serve two people, cooked as described below and sliced for serving.

2 kid spleens (or from other sources, in proportion); 5 cloves garlic, sliced; 1 dessertspoon thyme; 1 dessertspoon chopped basil; 3 tablespoons olive oil; the juice of 1 lemon

Wash the spleen, drain well and with a sharp knife open the small holes in the spleen and insert the sliced garlic.

Prepare a mixture of lemon juice, oil and herbs, and brush some of this over the spleens. Grill on a gentle heat, basting from time to time with the remaining oil, lemon and herb mixture.

The spleen is cooked when pricking produces no red liquid. Serve with grilled vegetables.

SPLEEN IN TOMATO SAUCE

Serves four

8 kid or lamb spleens; 5 ripe tomatoes, peeled and finely chopped; 1 wineglass white wine; 1½ dessertspoons chopped thyme; 1½ dessertspoons chopped parsley; 1 clove garlic; 1 large onion, finely chopped; 4 tablespoons olive oil

Wash and drain the spleens, prick them and rub in the herbs and a little garlic.

Place the chopped tomatoes and onions with four slices of garlic in a pan and cook for 15 minutes. Add the wine, simmer for 10 minutes and then pour in a cup of warm water.

Allow to cook for 1 minute more, then add the spleens. Cover with liquid, adding more water if necessary. Simmer until only a thick sauce remains.

MAGIRITSA

Traditionally, this is the first meal eaten after Lent. It is based on the intestines, stomach, liver, kidneys, heart and spleen of a lamb. Kid may be substituted if preferred and available. This recipe serves eight to ten.

Lamb or kid stomach, intestines, liver, lungs, kidneys, spleen and heart; 1 dessertspoon chopped dill; 1 dessertspoon chopped parsley; 5 spring onions, chopped; 2 cloves garlic, chopped; juice of 2 lemons; 6 tablespoons olive oil

First wash all the organs thoroughly. To clean the intestines, cut them lengthwise, then soak and wash the resulting material in water with the juice of several lemons squeezed into it.

Dice all meat ingredients into 1 cm cubes, then place in a large, shallow saucepan with all the remaining ingredients apart from the lemon juice. Cover with water and allow to simmer until most of the water has evaporated. Then add the lemon juice and stir gently. Cook for 1 minute more, then serve warm with vegetables of choice.

BRAIN

Stone Age people ate the brains and bone marrow of animals. These are still a delicacy in many countries.

DEER OR CALF BRAIN

Cook the brain until tender in water with a little salt substitute and 1–2 dessertspoons vinegar. Drain well and grill until browned.

When cooked, cover with a mixture of 2 tablespoons of olive oil, the juice of 1 lemon, and 1 dessertspoon chopped oregano. Serve either as a main course with vegetables or as a side dish.

Serves two as a main course, four as a side dish.

BRAIN AND CUCUMBERS

Serves two as a main course, four as a starter

Brain of calf or deer; 4 cucumbers; 1 wineglass vegetable stock; ¼ teaspoon ground cumin; 1 teaspoon honey; ½ teaspoon celery seeds; 1 dessertspoon olive oil; 2 egg yolks; black pepper

Boil the brain for 20 minutes, then allow to cool and dice. Slice the cucumbers lengthwise and place in a saucepan with the precooked, diced brain, the stock, honey, cumin, celery seeds and oil. Bring to the boil and simmer until the cucumbers are lightly cooked. Add the well-beaten yolks to bind the ingredients and sprinkle on black pepper. Serve either as a starter or with vegetables as a main course.

These recipes are only examples, there are many other ways in which game and organ meats can be brought into everyday use with no special skills. These foods should be complemented by a wide variety of vegetables, both cultivated and wild. Ample material is available for those interested in expanding their knowledge as to the use of vegetables in cooking, but few good books exist on the subject of wild vegetables. One which is recommended is *Eat the Weeds* by Ben Charles Harris (Keats, 1973).

WILD VEGETABLES

Wild vegetables have particular qualities and values. Among the commonest, and found easily in most environments, are dandelions, nettles, mustard greens and comfrey. These should be washed thoroughly, and then boiled or steamed until tender. Boiling seldom takes more than 2 to 3 minutes, and as little water as possible should be used. All are rich in vitamin C and minerals.

Once the vegetables are cooked and drained, place them in a bowl and dress with lemon juice and olive oil. Serve with crushed or thinly sliced raw garlic to accompany meat or a vegetarian meal.

Dandelions (*taraxacum officiale*) have a bitterness which is an acquired taste and only the leaves should be used. Eaten in small quantities, together with vegetarian savoury food or meat, they can be delicious. Basil added in cooking improves the flavour. If boiled, the water should be retained and drunk later, warm or cold, with added lemon juice to taste. This is rich in minerals and acts as a detoxifying liquid with strong diuretic properties. The young shoots can also be used raw in salads.

Only the tender young shoots of nettle (*urtica dioica*) should be picked. These are best eaten boiled or stewed. Another wild vegetable which can be safely consumed is chicory (*chicorium intybus*), also known as wild endive or blue sailor. This has lovely blue flowers in the early spring. The leaves may be eaten raw or steamed for just a few minutes, and served with lemon juice and olive oil.

Burdock (*atricum lapa*) is another wild delicacy. The young leaves are eaten and also the first year's stems. These can be steamed like asparagus and dressed with lemon juice. The young leaves should be collected in the spring, and the stems in summer. Again the cooking water can be consumed as a healthy drink.

There are numerous other edible wild plants, and seeking and eating these will pay dividends in terms of the variety of tasty, nutritious and inexpensive additions to diet that they provide.

SALT SUBSTITUTE FROM HERBS

There are various herbs which can be picked, and their dried
leaves powdered as a salt substitute. Among these are wild
carrot, yellow dock, golden rod, lambsquarter fruits, nettles,
peppergrass leaves and fruits, peppermint, sassafras leaves
and bark, shepherd's purse leaves and fruits, spearmint leaves
and young leaves of tansy.

These should be collected, and the whole plant hung in an
airy place to dry (not in the sun or there will be a loss of colour
and flavour). Then the dried leaves and/or berries can be
collected. Mixed together and powdered by a coffee mill,
processor, or in a mortar, they should then be sieved through
a cheese cloth to remove any coarse pieces of stem. One
dessertspoon of this powder together with two of kelp powder
(seaweed), which is available from health stores, and a teaspoon
of any mixture of powdered basil, celery seed, dill seed,
marjoram or thyme, will make a fine salt substitute, which
may be used directly on food, or in cooking.

REFERENCES

1. S. Boyd Eaton and Melvin Konner, 'Paleolithic Nutrition: A Consideration of its Nature and Current Implications', *New England Journal of Medicine*, January 1985, Vol. 312 No. 5, 283–9
2. E. Cheraskin and W. Ringsdorf, *Diet and Disease*, Keats, 1977 Jeffrey Bland, *Medical Application of Clinical Nutrition*, Keats, 1984
3. Jeffrey Bland, *Your Personal Health Programme*, Thorsons, 1983
4. Robert Coates, 'What is a Natural Diet?', *Nutrition and Health*, Vol. 1, 1982
5. Melvin Page, *Degeneration/Regeneration*, Biochemical Research Foundation, 1965
6. Weston Price, *Nutrition and Physical Degeneration*, Price-Pottenger Nutrition Foundation, 1937, reprinted 1971
7. Michael and Sheilagh Crawford, *What We Eat Today*, Neville Spearman, 1972
8. S. Boyd Eaton and Melvin Konner, *op.cit.*
9. Stewart Trusswell, 'ABC of Nutrition', *British Medical Journal*, 23 November 1985
10. Herbert Shelton, *Orthotrophy*, Health Research, California, 1956
11. S. Boyd Eaton and Melvin Konner, *op.cit.*
12. John Robson, *Journal of Human Nutrition*, February 1978
13. S. Boyd Eaton and Melvin Konner, *op.cit.*
14. C. Wells, *Bones, Bodies and Diseases*, Thames and Hudson, 1964
15. P. A. Janssems, *Paleopathology, Diseases and Injuries of Prehistoric Man*, John Baker, 1970
16. Robert Coates, 'What is a Natural Diet?', *Nutrition and Health*, Vol. 1 No. 1, 1982
17. Richard Dawkins, *The Selfish Gene*, Oxford University Press, 1976
18. Gerald Hirsch, 'Spontaneous Mutations Balance Reproductive Selective Advantage and Genetically Determined Longevity', *Mech. Ageing Dev.*, 9, 1979, 335–367
19. Richard Cutler, 'Evolution of Human Longevity, and the Genetic Complexity Governing Ageing Rate', *Proceedings of The National Academy of Science, USA*, 72(11), 1975, 4664–4668
20. Desmond Morris, *The Naked Ape*, Corgi Books, 1972
21. Lyall Watson, *Lightening Bird*, Hodder and Stoughton
22. Carleton Coon, *The Origin of the Races*, Jonathan Cape, 1968
23. Lyall Watson, *op.cit.*
24. Clark and Piggott, *Prehistoric Society*, Penguin, 1985
25. Jon Wynne-Tyson, *Food for a Future*, Abacus, 1975
26. Linus Pauling, *Vitamin C, the Common Cold and the Flu*, W. H. Freeman and Co., San Francisco, 1976
27. Herbert Shelton, *op.cit.*
28. Desmond Morris, *op.cit.*
29. Robert Coates, *op.cit.*
30. S. Boyd Eaton and Melvin Konner, *op.cit.*
31. Rudolph Ballentyne, *Diet and Nutrition, A Holistic Approach*, Himalayan International Institute, Pennsylvania, 1978
32. William Kelley, *One Answer to Cancer*, Kelley Foundation, 1974
33. Henry Bieler, *Diet is Your Best Medicine*, Bantam Books, 1978
34. Miriam Polunin, *The Right Way to Eat*, Granada Books, 1978
35. Barbara Wood, *The Economist*, 2 November 1974

36. Kenneth Mellanby, *Can Britain Feed Itself?*, Merlin Press, 1975
37. Roger Williams, *Biochemical Individuality*, University of Texas Press, 1976
38. Rudolph Ballentyne, *op.cit.*
39. Gary Null, *New Vegetarian*, Delta Books, 1978
40. Ruth Harrison, *Animal Machines*, Vincent Stuart, London, 1964
41. F. Paradisi et al, 'Is Fast Food Toxic?' *New England Journal of Medicine*, Vol. 313, No. 17, 1985, 1092
42. Michael and Sheilagh Crawford, *op.cit.*
43. Arne Dahlqvist, 'Lactose Intolerance', *Nutrition Abstracts and Reviews*, August 1984, 649–658
44. J. Brand et al, 'Lactose Malabsorption in Australian Aboriginal Children', *American Journal of Clinical Nutrition*, March 1985, 620–2
45. Arne Dahlqvist, *op.cit.*
46. F. Simoons, 'A Geographic Approach to Senile Cataracts. Possible Link with Milk Consumption', *Digestive Diseases and Sciences*, Vol. 27 No. 3, 1982, 257–64
47. Robert Coates, *op.cit.*
48. F. A. Oski, 'Is Bovine Milk a Health Hazard?' *Paediatrics*, 725, 1985, 182–5
49. S. Boyd Eaton and Melvin Konner, *op.cit.*
50. Linus Pauling, *op.cit.*
51. *Ibid.*
52. *Ibid.*
53. Roger Williams, *op. cit.*
54. Linus Pauling, *op.cit.*
55. Irwin Stone, *The Healing Factor: Vitamin C Against Disease*, Grosset and Dunslap, New York, 1972
56. Rudolph Ballentyne, *op.cit.*
57. E. Cheraskin and W. Ringsdorf, *op.cit.*
58. T. Basu and C. Schorah, *Vitamin C in Health and Disease*, Croom Helm, 1981
59. Desmond Morris, *op.cit.*
60. Granville Knight, *Clinical Ecology*, Charles Thomas, 1978
61. Weston Price, *op.cit.*
62. Robert McCarrison, *Nutrition and Health*, Faber & Faber, 1953
63. L. Jensen, *Man's Food*, Garrard Press, 1953
64. Desmond Morris, *op.cit.*
65. Denis Burkitt, *Refined Carbohydrate Foods and Disease*, Academic Press, 1975
66. Andrew Stanway, *Taking the Rough with the Smooth*, Pan, 1976
67. Rudolph Ballentyne, *op.cit.*
68. *Ibid.*
69. Stewart Trusswell, *op.cit.*
70. John Yudkin, *Pure, White and Deadly*, Davis-Poynter, 1972
71. S. Boyd Eaton and Melvin Konner, *op.cit.*
72. Jeffrey Bland, *Your Personal Health Programme*, *op.cit.*
73. S. Boyd Eaton and Melvin Konner, *op.cit.*
74. *Ibid.*
75. E. Cheraskin and W. Ringsdorf, *op.cit.*
76. Boris Chaitow, *A Timely Warning to a Sick Society*, Monograph, 1977
77. John Edwards, *The Roman Cookery of Apicius*, Rider, 1984

ABOUT THE AUTHOR

Leon Chaitow, ND, DO, MBNOA, is a well-known and respected nutritionist and osteopath.

He writes a regular column for *Here's Health*, Britain's leading health magazine, is a consultant editor and feature writer for the *Journal of Alternative Medicine*, and has contributed to several other magazines and journals including *Alternative Medicine Today* and *Vogue*.

He lectures all over the world and has written fifteen other books on nutrition and alternative medical methods.

Leon Chaitow gave up full-time practice in 1983 to concentrate on writing and now lives with his wife and daughter in Corfu.